# International Perspectives on Education Reform
Gita Steiner-Khamsi, Editor

Institutionalizing Health and Education for All

Global Goals, Innovations, and Scaling Up

Colette Chabbott
with Mushtaque Chowdhury

Foreword by Francisco O. Ramirez

Teachers College
Columbia University
New York and London

Published by Teachers College Press, 1234 Amsterdam Avenue, New York, NY
10027

Chapter 3 is a modified version of Chabbott, C. (2007). Carrot soup, magic bullets
and scientific research for education and development. *Comparative Education
Review, 51*(1), 71–94.

The 2nd part of Chapter 6 is a modified version of Chabbott, C. (2008). BRAC
goes global. In L. Chisholm & G. Steiner-Khamsi (Eds.), *South-south: Educational
development among equals?* (pp. 192–209). New York, NY: Teachers College Press.

Library of Congress Cataloging-in-Publication Data is available at loc.gov

ISBN 978-0-8077-5608-9 (paper)
ISBN 978-0-8077-7344-4 (ebook)

Printed on acid-free paper
Manufactured in the United States of America

22 21 20 19 18 17 16 15   8 7 6 5 4 3 2 1

Contents

Foreword

Institutionalizing Health and Education for All is that rare book, one that is grounded in decades of policy experiences in the international development field yet is also theoretically motivated. The former is evident in the richness of the detail in the comparative assessments of health and educational innovations in less-developed countries, especially Bangladesh. Colette Chabbott clearly inhabits the world of development organizations and professionals, and ultimately identifies with global health and educational goals. But she also understands that the institutionalization of these global goals and how they are to be attained create not only opportunities but also constraints on actors and action. This outlook uses and extends the world society perspective to make sense of similarities and differences in the health and education sectors from the viewpoint of all the relevant players. In doing so, this book avoids both an uncritical celebration of development work as well as its equally uncritical demonization.

This is not a "who done it" mystery novel. So it is reasonable to read the introductory and concluding chapters before turning to the case studies. The introduction is an essential roadmap, without which one could get lost in the trials and tribulations of never-ending reforms. But it is much more than a clear statement of the issues each chapter will address—it is a theorizing introduction that emphasizes the centrality and pervasiveness of world models of development and their associated policy blueprints. These models and blueprints are summarized as propositions (see Figure 1.1). The key thesis is that "Western Enlightenment" values and identities are privileged—e.g., education is the key to individual and national development. Success at both the individual and national levels is to be attained and gauged through rational/technical means anchored in the authority of science. Not surprisingly, much loose coupling takes place as reforms are imagined to be context-free, but alas, context matters. What it takes to look externally legitimate is often inconsistent with what is locally feasible, and at times, desirable.

This is a major issue throughout this book and one revisited in the Conclusions chapter. Context here refers not only to national and sub-national contexts, but also to organizational and sector contexts. Chabbott raises the question, "Can education learn from health?", and offers a nuanced answer: "Yes, but not blindly." Health crises command greater concern and resources from the international community; Primary School Student Retention does not arouse as much attention as Child Survival. Moreover, the science underlying health interventions is highly developed. But the underfunded and more uncertain educational field is more vulnerable to external legitimacy pressures that favor particular reforms, regardless of their efficacy. Some of the favored reforms ran counter to the taken-for-granted assumption that states should be in charge of schools. This complicates matters, especially for those who think of schools in de-politicized terms. There are cross-sector similarities, but also differences.

Chabbott also emphasizes the positive impact of trial-and-error user research in past health reforms, and argues that more of this type of research is needed in the ongoing early reading educational innovations. But here she confronts a second major issue: the unintended negative effect of accountability regimes that want evidence of success, and they want it yesterday. These regimes command center stage, and today's professionals are less field-savvy and more attuned to short-term (some would say short-sighted) scalable results. The new funding sources are less than patient. The institutional memory about how much trial and error took place in order to produce successful health reforms is fading. Learning from failures is not happening. This is not a promising situation.

But like Sisyphus, Chabbott is committed to moving the development boulder up the global hill. Much of the last chapter identifies factors that facilitate the climb, from characteristics of context that facilitate scaling innovations, to features of innovations that aid launching and sustaining global initiatives. Here and there Chabbott flashes a knuckle in the direction of her fellow development professionals, noting, for instance, that they complain about the rigidity of bureaucrats without displaying any awareness of their own disciplinary blinders. But there are no devils in this narrative about international development as a field. Experts and organizations are often trapped by blueprints that, if slavishly adhered to, will lead to throwing away the babies with the bath water. This book champions a healthy pragmatism in the pursuit of educational reform: Focus on what works. It challenges the universalism that fuels impatience with context-contingent reforms. Ironically, both pragmatism and universalism have standing in the wider world culture. Aligning these different principles to generate better practice is indeed a challenge.

This book offers many examples of how the universalistic authority of science can be linked to local realities in order to produce successful reforms. There are success stories, like how oral therapy education emerged and was scaled "out of the basket and into the world." And there are hopeful beginnings, like the rise and effort to institutionalize early-grades reading. But, however committed, Chabbott is not sanguine about the development boulder. Neither should we.

—Francisco O. Ramirez

Acknowledgments

Francisco O. Ramirez and John W. Meyer of Stanford University for new eyes and fresh ways of using them. And for demonstrating that when it starts getting absurd, we may well be on the right track.

Nancy Kendall, who is a perennial source of new and intriguing ideas, a tireless writing partner, and a bottomless source of optimism.

David and Jean Sack, who opened their home, introduced me to the history of ICDDR,B, and invited me to think about what education might learn from health.

The staff of the BRAC Nonformal Primary Education Program, particularly Kaniz Fatema, Erum Marium, Safiqul Islam, and Nashida Ahmed.

James Williams and colleagues at the International Education Program at George Washington University, who have given a part-time academic a full-time home.

Gita Steiner-Khamsi, for her patience with my process and for reminding us that the Cold War mattered.

The late Catherine H. Lovell, for beginning to lay down a trail of crumbs to guide us through the complex organization that is BRAC.

My husband, Theodore H. Thomas, who helped generate many of the ideas here and who was (largely) stoic throughout the three-year detour from our previously interesting life that this book entailed. Okay. Some fun now.

SOURCES AND READERS

In addition to the documents and personal communications cited throughout the book, dozens of individuals were generous with their bookshelves, their experiences, and their time. Nonetheless, they are not responsible for any errors in these chapters, nor do they necessarily agree with the analysis in the chapters with which I have associated them below.

Chapter 2: Margaret Sutton, interviewee No. 1 in 1993 who got the snowball rolling on EFA research. For critical eyes: Patricia Weiss Fagen, Rebecca Rhodes, and Sheila Barry Tacon. Chapter 3: William Greenough

III, Richard Cash, John and Candy Rohde, Robert and Quincy Northrup, David Nalin, David Sachar, Henry and Bunny Mosley, Charlene Dale Riikonen, Norbert Hirschhorn, and David Sachar. For critical eyes: David Post, Mark Ginsburg, and several anonymous reviewers when a version of this chapter was submitted to the *Comparative Education Review* and later appeared in the February 2007 issue.

Chapters 4 and 5: Fazle H. Abed, Manzoor Ahmed, Saleuddin Ahmed, Aminul Alam, Arif Anwar, Chitra Ayar, Samdani Fakir, Kaniz Fatema, Sunil K. Ghosh, Khondaker Ariful Islam, Safiqul Islam, Andrew Jenkins, Md. Monwar Hossain Khadaker, Erum Mariam, Saeeda Anis Prew, Ian Smiley, Graham White. For critical eyes: David Post, Mark Ginsburg, and several anonymous reviewers who wisely rejected earlier versions of the last half of Chapter 5.

Chapter 6: Tapan Kumar Acharjee, Rubana Afroz, Shahabuddin Ahmed, Md. Hanif Ali, Mizan-ur-Rahman Chowdhury, Cooper Dawson, Cole Dodge, Tajul Islam, James Jennings, Peter Laugharn, Sarah Kahando, Rashida Parveen, Mima Parisic, Abdul Rahman, Milton Roy, Marc Sommers, and A. K. M. Kamal Uddin. For critical eyes: Gita Steiner-Khamsi, Linda Chisholm, and an anonymous reviewer of the second half of this chapter when it was accepted for publication in L. Chisholm & G. Steiner-Khamsi (Eds.) (2008). *South-South: Educational Development Among Equals?* New York: Teachers College Press.

Chapter 7: Helen Abadzi, Anita Anastasio, Laila Apnan Banu, Penelope Bender, Rachel Carnegie, Luis Crouch, Shoaib Danish, Amy Jo Dowd, Amber Gove, Clarence Malone, Chloe O'Gara, and Helen Stannard. Jane Benbow, who commissioned the first paper for USAID on early grades reading, Chabbott, C. (2006). "Accelerating Early Grades Reading in High Priority EFA Countries: A Desk Review." Washington, DC: USAID/American Institutes for Research. Amber Gove, who commissioned Chabbott, C. (2010). "Social Mobilization to Promote & Support Early Literacy." Washington, DC: Research Triangle Institute. (Unpublished. Available on EGR Community of Practice website.)

Institutionalizing Health and Education for All

CHAPTER 1

Introduction

Science and the technological innovation it produces are pivotal to modern conceptions of national and international progress and socioeconomic development. Indeed, innovations in medicine, agriculture, and structural engineering, among other fields, have made possible more radical improvements in the lives of more human beings in the past hundred years than could have been imagined in the previous millennium. At the time of the United Nations' 1978 Health for All (HFA) and 1990 Education for All (EFA) declarations, innovations were expected to play an equally important role in global efforts to secure universal access to both basic health care and basic education in the space of a decade or two.

For many in the international development community, some of whom played significant roles in constructing, promoting, and implementing global goals, progress toward these goals has been disappointing. Several analyses at the end of the first decades for HFA and EFA concluded that the amount of funding mobilized fell far short of needs. They further concluded that government willpower to undertake the radical changes necessary to bring about dramatic changes in a decade or two rarely materialized. The Millennium Development Goals (MDGs) promulgated following the United Nations Millennium Summit of 2000 consequently incorporated narrower health and education goals, largely focused on children, to be achieved by 2015. By 2012, with even these narrower formulations still beyond reach, far from abandoning the global goals, the international development community was already constructing new goals for the post-2015 period.

ON THE SAME TRACK, AT DIFFERENT SPEEDS

This book explores the persistence of the global goals blueprint in the last quarter of the 20th and the first quarter of the 21st centuries as a phenomenon driven by organizations in the international development field. The world society perspective, described in greater detail below, serves both to conceptualize this field and to study its variable impact on the formulation and implementation of global initiatives in health and education. Much of the variance may relate to the more sophisticated Western science mobilized to support health initiatives, as well as greater professionalization throughout the health sector. In contrast, education is more of a nation-state–led enterprise, more closely linked to national culture than health is. This explains, in part, why innovations are more readily adapted and diffused in health than in education.

Several chapters aim at global or international analyses, and others focus on activities in Bangladesh, a country that is an exemplary site for studying the workings of the international development field. Not incidentally, Bangladesh was also the site where two interventions that played important roles in HFA and EFA were invented, adapted, and diffused nationally and then internationally. These closely related case studies, which comprise the next six chapters, document the processes involved as:

- international development organizations *imagined* HFA and EFA at the global level in fundamentally similar and comprehensive, and later in more selective, terms (Chapter 2);
- scientists working in one international research center *invented* one innovation that helped to inspire the Child Survival initiative (Chapter 3);
- a single national relief and development organization *adapted* and *scaled up* that health innovation, closely related to HFA, and did the same for an innovation in education, similarly related to EFA, about a decade apart in one country (Chapters 4 and 5);
- those same scientists and that same organization *scaled out* the health and the education innovations *to other countries* (Chapter 6); and
- international development professionals designed and tried to use an innovative measure of education quality to *reimagine* and *promote* new, selective global education goals (Chapter 7).

These case studies show that the failure to date to achieve global goals in health and education is not solely a function of inadequate funding, willpower, or time. Rather, cultural and organizational factors in world society encouraged expansive approaches to global goals and, at the same time, constrained the ability of governments and international organizations to recognize and fund technologies that might have achieved the goals. Some constraints arose as the international development organizations involved at many stages of global goal construction and implementation misconceived the process by which innovations capable of achieving global goals take form and scale-up.

Many of those misconceptions derived logically from models, blue-prints, scripts, and identities[1] that the international development field itself constructed over the last 50 years to rationalize its own activities. These rationalizations derived from another time and place, for example, from Western Enlightenment notions of progress and justice, and emerged piece-meal in response to a variety of crises and contingencies. Nonetheless, over time they have become amalgamated into a compelling model of "develop-ment" and institutionalized in the structuring documents of governments and international organizations. By the end of the 20th century, this model of reality had taken on a life of its own, projecting itself as a coherent body of knowledge, demanding that international activities of all types and sizes conform to it.

The impact of international development models and scripts on the global goals blueprint is immediately apparent in the origins of EFA. From the earliest discussions, EFA was patterned on HFA, despite clear, obviously deep differences in the science undergirding the health and education sec-tors, such as:

- types and levels of empiricism,
- the size of the units of analysis,
- the universality of findings,
- the number of specialties and subspecialties, and
- the length of time and precision with which intervention outcomes can be measured.

As a result of these factors, in 1978 the health sector had a small stock-pile of universal, stand-alone interventions with the capacity to speed the realization of selective global goals and a critical mass of professionals ready to pursue such goals. In contrast, the education sector in 1990 remained locked into a much more complex institutionalized model of mass schooling committed to much broader and more diverse goals, all of which discour-aged the development of universal, stand-alone education interventions.

CAN EDUCATION LEARN SOMETHING FROM HEALTH?

Despite these significant differences, the health sector's longer experience and greater success in producing innovations capable of advancing global goals—for better or worse—hold many interesting and relevant insights for scholars and practitioners studying or promoting global goals for educa-tion. A cross-sectoral analysis can help to correct the tendency to attribute many inconsistencies and conceptual conflicts to EFA and its successors, rather than to the international development field. In addition, comparing a health and an education innovation emerging in the same country, from the same organization, reduces the contextual "noise" typical in existing cross-national studies of educational innovation.[2] Finally, by comparing innovations that emerged a decade or more apart in the same context, these case studies capture some of the increasing rigidity in international development blueprints and scripts over time that make implementing initiatives in education more problematic than earlier initiatives in health.

Official reports issued by international development organizations constitute an important source for these case studies, as do interviews with staff in those organizations. The reports tend to frame the organizations' actions in terms of rational decisionmaking in response to new technologies and funding, largely independent of their historical or organizational context. In contrast, staffs in those organizations describe a more complex story full of individual agency, budget constraints, corrupt governments and organizations, and heroic efforts to accomplish something in a decade or less. The case studies in this volume, therefore, recognize the roles of scientists, development workers, and international development organizations both as individuals and as collectivities, enacting and acting on identities determined by the environments—global, national, organizational, physical—in which they are embedded. For example, at the most basic, geographic level, scientists and field workers involved in the discovery of oral rehydration at a research center in Bangladesh insisted that a scientific laboratory located in an environment awash with cholera patients and epidemics produced better research questions and faster innovations than would have been the case had the center been located elsewhere. Even so, the process was not fast. In the case of oral rehydration, the time span from the founding of an international research center dedicated to cholera research to the development of an effective, large-scale, locally appropriate cholera treatment was almost 20 years. These case studies, therefore, describe processes lasting 3 to 5 or even 10 years, much longer than those typically funded by individual international development organizations.

Inventions emerging from scientific research centers rarely have direct impact on global goals. Almost always the inventions must be adapted to field conditions and expanded on a limited basis before they can be scaled up nationally. Moreover, the case studies suggest that much of this process must be repeated in each new context, and that one country may comprise several, sometimes dozens of, contexts, depending on the nature of the innovation. At each step in the innovation process, new problems arise and require addressing through trial and error. At any step, therefore, the innovation may be perceived as failing. Over time, however, the discourse in the international development community in which potential development funders are embedded has tolerated less and less failure. Rather, it has pressed for large-scale results in the time frame of the typical project cycle, 3 to 5 years or a decade at most. Each of the cases in Chapters 4 through 6, therefore, identifies characteristics of the innovation as well as organizational and contextual factors that affect the quality and speed of the *diffusion of innovations* (Wejnert, 2002).

Two sociological perspectives inform discussions of the nature and diffusion of the two innovations throughout this book. Everett C. Rogers' *Diffusion of Innovations* (2003, p. 19) provided the broadest definition of an innovation: "an idea, practice, or object [or some combination of these three] that is perceived as new by an individual [or unit of adoption]." Rogers also provided the concept of *relational* diffusion, a person-to-person process demanding significant personal leadership and agency. In contrast, the notion of *institutional* diffusion or isomorphism, the process by which similar (iso-) forms (-morph) diffuse across space and time, somewhat independent of their technical merits, draws on Paul J. DiMaggio and Walter W. Powell (DiMaggio & Powell, 1983) at the organizational level and on the work of John W. Meyer (Strand & Meyer, 2009/1993), Francisco O. Ramirez (Ramirez & Boli, 1987), and their students at the global or world society level. One of Meyer's major contributions to the diffusion literature was the notion that, in addition to activities, ideas, practices, and objects, theories play an important role in the speed at which innovations are adopted. For example, Meyer (Meyer, 1977) referred to education as a theory of knowledge and of personnel. Knowledge counts if it is anchored in education; nutritional science boosts chicken soup from folk medicine to real science, and certified nutritional scientists boost confidence in the finding that chicken soup really is good for you.[3]

Although sometimes portrayed as conflicting, the relational and institutional diffusion literatures intersect at the point where individuals or groups attempt to place an innovation on a more secure, long-term footing, not dependent on further human agency, that is, to *institutionalize* it. According to DiMaggio (1988), creating an institution, something that has become so taken for granted that it no longer needs human agency to sustain it, paradoxically requires a good deal of personal agency. Rogers identifies five categories of actors in the diffusion process: innovators, early adopters, early majority, late majority, and laggards. In the cases in this book, therefore, individual "norm entrepreneurs" or carriers (Finnemore & Sikkink, 1998) fall into the first two categories. To the extent they are successful, over time, their ideas became institutionalized and carried by the organizations in which these individuals were embedded.

In addition to offering new directions for scholarly research, this perspective also aims to provide professionals in international development,

particularly those practicing in the education sector, with a better understanding of the blueprints, scripts, and identities that constrain and amplify
their activities in order to better build on or subvert them. As described in
these cases, many of the quirks, externalities, and dysfunctions the actors
experience are not unique to one or two organizations or even to the field of
international development organizations. Rather, they are typical of organizations operating in fields with specific characteristics, including eminently
profitable organizations, such as General Electric and Disney, as well as successful nonprofits, such as hospitals and art museums.

FRAMEWORK AND CONSTRUCTS

Six chapters constitute the body of the book, bookended by this introduction and by a final chapter that offers summary reflections on the book and
some potential directions for practitioners and researchers who remain interested in the global goals phenomenon. The cases laid out in these chapters
all point to the importance of science and measurement in rendering some
innovations more universal and harder to resist than others. Clearly many
health interventions are legitimated by natural sciences, such as microbiology and virology, and come closer to being universal than does a particular approach to teaching phonics or long division. Furthermore, Cole and
Ramirez (2013) found a greater sense of urgency around respecting rights
having to do with physical integrity, such as freedom from torture, than
around rights that relate to civil and political rights, such as free speech.
Along similar lines, rights to health are more closely associated with physical welfare—mortality, morbidity—and may be more widely respected and
similarly interpreted than rights to education. Crises in health are simply
taken more seriously than crises in education.

Many of the insights offered in this book emerged by bringing a world
society perspective to bear on both scholarly and practitioner notions about
education for development. Ramirez (2012) explained that world society
scholars first engaged in a question of vital interest to comparative education scholars in the 1980s: Why did nation-state after nation-state expand
mass education after World War II? He concluded:

> (i) Nation-states acquire legitimacy to the degree that they enact proper nation-
> state identity; (ii) the expansion of education is a central feature of the enactment
> of proper nation-state identity; and thus (iii) nation-states expand schooling be-
> yond what one might expect if increased schooling were simply a reaction to
> local or national conditions. (p. 426)

Ramirez and Boli (1987) argued that nation-states, no less than individuals and organizations, are embedded in an environment, a world society, that makes some choices seem more rational and some experts more authoritative than others. The world society perspective is part of a larger neo-institutionalist approach that asks why certain ideas and ways of organizing action, once in place, may become taken for granted as the natural order of things, that is, become *institutionalized* (Berger & Luckmann, 1967). Establishing or dismantling an institution often requires much interest and agency on the part of self-conscious actors (DiMaggio, 1988), but once the change is in place, the logic that animated the actors may become invisible and immutable to those who inherit that institution.

For example, we tend to forget the relatively recent reification of modern individuals, organizations, and nation-states. For most of human history, traditional collectivities—family, tribe, clan, or religious community—not individuals, were the primary actors. The notions that individuals had rights somewhat independent of their membership in such traditional collectivities and that those individuals could organize to pursue some common, rational goal, more or less independent of those collectivities, are relatively recent ideas (Thomas, Meyer, Ramirez, & Boli, 1987). The modern, goal-driven rather than relationship-driven organization made up of individual members and the modern, sovereign nation-state constituted of individual citizens, with borders determined somewhat independent of ethnicity or clan, are both less than 500 years old.

The Western Enlightenment gave rise to the concept of universal individual human rights, an innovation in ethics codified at the international level less than 50 years ago[4] (Drori, Meyer, & Hwang, 2006). Since that time, human rights have been rapidly incorporated as timeless in international covenants, national constitutions, and school curricula (Suarez, 2007). That schooling is one of those universal human rights and that schools serve as the principal means to prepare future citizens and workers to participate as equals in the modern nation-state and the modern economy, and that this should occur somewhat independent of their immediate forebears' stations in life, are, likewise, recent notions. Finally, the notion that wealthier nation-states, sometimes independent of their economic and security interests, should find it in their interest to help poorer nation-states develop their economies and the general welfare of their citizens is less than 100 years old. A field of organizations to promote such notions only emerged in the last 50 years.

World society scholars argue that forgetting the recent provenance of institutions such as universal formal mass schooling and universal human rights is in part the result of the rise of a world culture. Every collectivity, traditional or modern—families, tribes, organizations, nations—over time develops a culture that can be studied through its artifacts. The artifacts take many forms: potsherds or grocery lists or applications for patents or school curricula, to name a few. The work of neo-institutional sociologists engaged in world society research explores the emergence of this new collectivity—the world society created when nation-states, organizations, and individuals interact at the global level—and the effects of the world culture that it is producing (Krucken & Drori, 2009; Meyer, Boli, Thomas, & Ramirez, 1997).

The means to achieve institutionalized ends at the global level, such as universal human rights or national socioeconomic development, may also, in and of themselves, become institutionalized. In the modern period, the Western scientific approach—empirical, quantitative, rational, driven by the experimental method[5]—has been the dominant norm governing legitimate means to public ends. This has resulted in a tendency in modern organizational fields and professions to resort to standardized technology using quantifiable, standardized inputs and outputs and to cloak ordinary work—which by nature involves a good amount of subjective, individual judgment—with a veneer of science. In this context, the term *technology* is used in its broadest sense: systematic actions designed to maximize effect at minimum cost (Ellul, 1964/1954). In a perfectly competitive market,[6] where inputs and outputs can be readily measured and all costs and transactions are transparent to all buyers and sellers, efficiency concerns naturally drive the standardization of technology. This is competitive isomorphism. In fields of endeavor where perfect market conditions do not pertain, three institutional forces nonetheless tend to generate standardization or isomorphism in technology and procedures. First, key buyers, suppliers, or investors force producers to do so; second, producers mimic other producers whom they regard as more successful; and/or third, professionals in that field establish "best practices" or norms (DiMaggio & Powell, 1983). Thus, both competitive and institutional isomorphism are involved in creating increasing conformity at various levels of many industries and fields.

INTERNATIONAL DEVELOPMENT AS AN INSTITUTION

The conditions for perfect competition clearly do not pertain in the international development field. This reduces opportunities for competition and brings institutional isomorphism of all types into play. First, dependence on scarce donor funding leads to much intentional and unintentional coercive isomorphism, conformity to donor norms, and formal operating procedures on the parts of recipient governments, grantees, and contractors. However, porous labor markets between international donors and international grant-ees and contractors are such that professionals moving from one organiza-tion to another in the course of their normal careers try to reduce ambiguity and dissonance by working with other professionals to establish common norms and standard operating procedures across the field. Finally, in the absence of coercion and professional norms, many organizations will try to achieve the success of leading organizations by copying their discourse and activities. Needless to say, all forms of institutional isomorphism contribute to significant loose coupling between what nation-states, organizations, and professionals say and what they do.

Thus, in the context of the current world culture, where rationality and the search for the "one best technology" drive the development of many activities, professionals emerge as pivotal actors in organizations and in the modern world polity. The current world culture authorizes professionals to take action based on some certified expertise not available to the general public (i.e., their jurisdiction), often acquired in formal higher education or certification programs (Abbott, 1988). Professionals may be scientists or managers working inside organizations or as external consultants to organizations; in all cases, their commitment to professional norms is ex-pected to be stronger than their commitment to any particular organization. These norms encourage professionals to think about themselves as actors, uniquely responsible for improving outcomes and efficiency in their juris-diction. At the global level, many professionals construct their identity as apolitical technicians committed to advancing progress independent of their nationality or personal interests and may band together to form epistemic communities that seek to influence policies both inside and outside their nation-state (Haas, 1992). As such, they establish standards, norms, bench-marks, blueprints, guidelines, and "best practices" based on the state of sci-ence in their jurisdictions. As individuals, these professionals may be more or less self-interested or altruistic, but to survive as professionals they must defend their jurisdiction.

Like most modern individuals, who have been socialized to think of themselves as independent actors assured of the efficacy of the standard technology in their field (if not always entirely convinced), development professionals place great faith in scientific innovation to remedy earlier problems and to accelerate future progress. This approach assumes that technological fixes exist for many problems and that where they don't, concerted, systematic effort can produce them in short order. As such, these professionals play an important role in diffusing innovations from the industrialized to the less industrialized world and sometimes within the less industrialized world. Beginning with the individual disease eradication campaigns of the 1950s, learning from the World Population Conferences of the 1960s and 1970s, by the end of the 20th century, professionals in the international development field had established a widely shared blueprint for the creation and pursuit of global goals through global conferences and campaigns.

For the purposes of this analysis, Figure 1.1 summarizes some propositions from the world society literature that are salient to the construction and promotion of global goals and of technological innovations as a key component in achieving them. At the end of several chapters, these propositions are translated into generalizations about organizations, innovations, and contexts relative to global development initiatives and goals. This effort to make generalizations is one feature that distinguishes comparative and historical social science from conventional historical case study approaches.

Figure 1.1. Propositions About World Society Relevant to Global Goals, Technological Innovation, and International Development Organizations

P1.1. Since the end of World War II, increased interaction at the global level among individuals, organizations, and nation-states has built up a "world society," which has led to the emergence of the current "world culture" and a host of new associations and organizations.

P1.2. The current world culture comprises individuals, organizations, and nation-states in terms consistent with Western Enlightenment norms, including rationality, individualism, professionalism, voluntarism, and global citizenship. This culture is neither the best nor likely the worst possible; rather, it is a reflection of the hegemony of Western science in commerce and in military affairs for at least the last 200 years.

P1.3. This world culture produces and diffuses models of reality, blueprints, identities, and scripts that circumscribe the legitimate activities of individuals, organizations, and nation-states, privileging those that conform to the Western Enlightenment notion of individual human rights and that claim science as the basis for rational decisionmaking.

P1.4. These Enlightenment notions and their corollary—that positive, planned action can accelerate the natural course of human progress—provided the raison d'être for the rise of a field of organizations to promote individual and national development.

    P1.4.1. This field of organizations gives rise to development professionals, who in turn shape the standards, norms, and best practices that shape the activities of those organizations.

    P1.4.2. Education occupies a privileged place in the imagining of international development.

P1.5. In international development organizations, the pride of place given to Western natural science leads to the privileging of explicit knowledge and quantitative data in constructing rational, carefully considered development

CASE SELECTION, SOURCES, AND METHODS

This book aims to make statements about the activities of international development organizations, international scientists and professionals, national nongovernmental organizations, South-South exchange/mutual development, and global goals. Three of the eight chapters, however, focus on just one country, Bangladesh, and those chapters, plus one of more international scope, concentrate on two organizations. For a book that claims to be of global interest, why this narrow focus?

First, Bangladesh is a quintessential product of the post-World War II global order. Following a cyclone that killed more than 500,000 people in 1970, a War of Independence from Pakistan in 1971 eliminated large numbers of intellectuals and senior government officers. At independence, Bangladesh's lack of natural resources beyond soil, water, and people; the

---

Figure 1.1. (continued)

plans and in describing development progress. At the same time, the Enlightenment's moral emphasis on the sanctity of the individual demands expedited responses by national governments and international organizations in times of humanitarian crisis. This emphasis on the individual also makes many types of inequality less palatable and increases demands for equitable development of a sort that would not occur naturally.

P1.5.1. Over time, standardized national data will be demanded in order to rationalize an increasing number of activities at the global level in terms of both progress and equity, particularly the activities of international development donors.

P1.6. Because these blueprints, identities, and scripts are constructed at the global level and privilege the Western Enlightenment, activities in contexts that have less contact with the global level or with Western Enlightenment values are likely to be loosely coupled with or decoupled from policy statements at the global or national level.

P1.7. With the advent of the Internet and of wireless communications, easier scrutiny by and comparisons with the larger world increase formal conformity across many different contexts. This in turn increases loose coupling or decoupling between global and local models, blueprints, identities, and scripts, which stimulates more scrutiny, with the same effects.

P1.8. Over time, the progressive nature of rationalization in the current world culture leads to increasing isomorphism in the categories and quantification of legitimate nation-state activities/qualities at the global level.

P1.9. World culture changes piecemeal. Change often demands significant human agency focused on a specific component. The resulting change is likely to take hold more quickly in contexts closely tied to the international community and more slowly in contexts at greater remove.

---

high frequency of cyclones, floods, and other natural disasters; and regular cholera epidemics and the persistence of smallpox led one undiplomatic U.S. diplomat to label the new country a "basket case."[7] Not surprisingly, in the 1970s GNP per capita in Bangladesh was among the lowest in the world, and a famine in 1974 led to about 1.5 million deaths, seeming to confirm the hopelessness of Bangladesh's situation.

Yet as soon as Bangladesh declared independence in 1971, a host of nation-state privileges and responsibilities were immediately conferred upon its fledgling government and the international community was obliged to support it. Since independence, the Bangladesh economy has grown and population growth has been significantly checked. Between 1970 and 2010 the mortality rate for children under 5 years old fell from 228 to 56.[8] Bangladesh is within reach of food self-sufficiency in some years, though income inequality and vulnerability to international price fluctuations means that millions live chronically hungry. All of this has been accomplished without charismatic or draconian authoritarian leadership, in spite of three military coups, several states of emergency, and some of the highest rates of corruption in the world. Bangladesh, therefore, is as difficult a development environment as any in the world. Whatever has been accomplished there cannot be exactly replicated in other low-income countries, but it represents a baseline for the realm of possibility.

Second, few senior Bangladeshi civil servants survived the War of Independence, severely restricting the government's ability to plan and effectively deliver routine human services and emergency relief to all areas of the country. Immediately following the war, therefore, leading international nongovernmental humanitarian and development organizations—CARE, Oxfam, Save the Children, Lutheran World Relief, World Vision, and Catholic Relief Services, among others—established offices in Dhaka, the capital, in the 1970s. Largely unconstrained by outside military or strategic interests in the first two decades of independence, and constrained fitfully by democratic governments since the 1990s, international development organizations, and the professionals within them, have had as much latitude in shaping development strategies and activities in Bangladesh as they have had anywhere in the world. All of these factors helped to make Bangladesh, at least until 2000, a microcosm of how the international development field works.

Third, within 15 years of independence, more than a thousand local nongovernmental organizations (NGOs) had formed and claimed to be doing humanitarian or development work in Bangladesh. From this fertile organizational environment two very large and effective NGOs stand out: Grameen Bank and BRAC, originally the Bangladesh Rehabilitation Assistance Committee. In time, BRAC adapted and scaled up two innovations that are among a handful frequently referred in both HFA (Child Survival) and EFA (Universal Primary Education) literature as promising innovations demonstrating that ambitious global goals could be met within a decade or two. BRAC presents a rare opportunity to study the process of innovation both in health and in education while holding constant both the organization and the context.

Fourth, the work of the Pak-SEATO Cholera Research Laboratory (f. 1961, PS-CRL, the Cholera Lab) and its later incarnation, the International Center for Diarrheal Disease Research, Bangladesh (f. 1978, ICDDR,B, the Diarrhea Center), offers a rare opportunity to look at the role science played in inventing an innovation that was central to the formulation of a global goal and to making rapid progress toward achieving it. Oral rehydration therapy was the product of modern microbiology research, highly legitimate science, conducted at the Cholera Research Laboratory; from there scientists helped to carry and adapt it to other countries. The education sector had no parallel to the Cholera Research Laboratory. Nonetheless, Chapter 3 explores some implications the Cholera Lab offers for EFA.

Finally, the details in this book should not encourage others to attempt to replicate the innovations described in other contexts. As Samoff and colleagues have written about scaling up innovations in Africa (Samoff, Sebatane, & Dembele, 2005), what perhaps needs to be replicated is not the innovation but the environment that allows for innovation through trial and error. The case studies, particularly those related to scaling up in Africa in Chapter 6, attempt to draw out what environmental factors might be particularly salient for expanding mass primary education in those countries with the farthest to go reach universal primary education (UPE). In addition, the accounts of both innovations described in this book place much emphasis on failures because they are so often left out of the accounts written by and for the international development community. Social scientists, in contrast, tend to learn more from falsification—from what doesn't work—than from "success."[9]

Sources

The material assembled to inform this analysis derives from both primary and secondary sources. The primary sources include first-person semi-structured interviews I conducted from 2003 to 2012 with principals in the development or implementation of the innovations of interest. Informants include current and former researchers at the Cholera Research Laboratory and its successor ICDDR,B, BRAC, and, to a lesser extent, UNICEF (United Nations Children's Fund). In addition to the usual peer-reviewed studies published in academic journals and doctoral dissertations, secondary sources include unpublished memoirs, as well as unpublished oral histories and published accounts featuring the principals or the principal organizations. For the principal organizations, I also draw on annual reports, websites, newsletters, and other published and unpublished reports. For Chapters 4 and 5, BRAC's Research and Evaluation Division's online database of its reports (1970s-present)[10] is a particularly valuable historical resource. Finally, because four chapters focus on national and local-level activities, several organizations central to the health and education sectors but which maintain a relatively small presence in Third World countries, such as WHO and UNESCO, are mainly addressed through secondary sources.

Access to much of this material and all of these informants was made possible by nearly 30 years of development work in Bangladesh, beginning with 4 years in full-time residence in the 1980s. Personal ties to leaders in BRAC, ICDDR,B, and UNICEF provided more insights into decision-making and cross-organizational ties between staff and funders than might have been possible otherwise. Finally, Chapter 7 is largely informed by papers and short-term consultancies on early-grade reading, the first commissioned by the American Institutes for Research in 2005, followed by work at the BRAC University Institute of Education, CARE, the Consultative Group for Early Childhood Care and Development, the William and Flora Hewlett Foundation, the Research Triangle Institute, and Save the Children.

A. Mushtaque R. Chowdhury was BRAC's first researcher, and he co-wrote the definitive history of BRAC's oral rehydration therapy program (Chowdhury & Cash, 1996). He has since served in many senior positions in the international public health community, including as visiting professor at the Mailman School of Public Health at Columbia University, representative for the Rockefeller Foundation in Asia, and founding dean of the James P. Grant School of Public Health at BRAC University. The abbreviated account of transforming oral rehydration salts into *lobon-gur* in Chapter 4 and of scaling up BRAC's oral rehydration therapy program in Chapter 5 draws heavily on his 1995 book, and he has reviewed and strengthened several versions of those chapters.

My position as a native English speaker, based at a large university located in Washington, D.C., provided easy access to bilateral development agencies based in the Anglophone world, particularly USAID, and also to international organizations with offices in the United States, such as UNICEF, the World Bank, and Save the Children. In addition, I have access to the country offices of those same agencies and many other national NGOs operating in Bangladesh. These organizations account for more than half of all international development aid for basic education, but by relying on them, my account of the workings of international development field likely reflects a mainstream bias. Away from the mainstream, other, more revolutionary things may be occurring, and I hope other researchers will come forward to help create a more complete, nuanced account of the process of setting global goals and mobilizing around them.

Finally, my perspective on measurement is strongly informed by 3 years at the National Research Council, where I directed a board that provided expert advice to the United States with respect to its participation in cross-national, large-scale studies of student achievement such as TIMSS, PISA, and PIRLS. My time at the NRC also overlapped with the NRC's differences with the George W. Bush administration's Department of Education with respect to three issues: Reading First, the establishment of an Institute of Education Sciences, and the role of randomized controlled trials in education research. All three issues figure significantly throughout this book.

Methods

The case studies are essentially insider, narrative accounts. In the interest of time and accessibility, I have refrained from detailed analyses of quantitative data uncovered in the course of writing, instead highlighting them at salient points in the text. These include, among others, BRAC Research and Evaluation Division's database of reports and publications; databases of innovations in education created by UNESCO and UNICEF; monitoring websites for various global initiatives; and the International Union of Associations' online database of nongovernmental organizations.

TERMINOLOGY AND ACRONYMS

Many common terms used in this book have a special meaning and a normative connotation in the context of international development. Putting quotation marks around every instance of these common words throughout the text would be tedious. This section provides the core meaning of those terms in the context of this analysis.

An *intervention* consists of a systematic action of one entity intended to affect another; an intervention may or may not be innovative. All interventions involve a *technology*—as defined earlier: systematic actions designed to maximize effect at minimum cost. Information and communication technologies are one well-known type of technology, but so are teaching methods, such as the Systematic Method for Reading Success developed at the University of California, Berkeley. All interventions take place in a *context* or *environment*, which are defined, in the context of this book, as the characteristics of setting external to the target of the intervention—i.e., individuals, organizations, or nation-states—that have the potential to shape effectiveness or salience. A *measure* provides the means to calculate the effectiveness of an intervention in a particular context. Different measures vary in their authoritativeness and in the degree of consensus they have achieved among professionals.

As noted earlier, an *innovation* is "an idea, practice, or object [or some combination of these three] that is perceived as new by an individual [or unit of adoption]" (Rogers & Shoemaker, 1971, p. 19). In the context of this book, an innovation may be of several types, and three are highlighted here. A *deliverable* is any service or product with which the client cannot readily supply himself or herself. A *delivery agent* is a person who is a primary point of contact between intended clients and the deliverable. A *delivery support system* comprises all the services supplied by the implementing organization necessary for delivery agents to operate effectively. In this analysis, the process of innovation comprises several steps, beginning with *imagining* some connection between global goals and interventions; *inventing* a product or service in one context; *adapting* an innovation effective in one context to another, similar context; *scaling up* an innovation proven effective in one context on a small scale to a larger scale; and *scaling out* an innovation proven successful on a large scale in one context to another context.

The Western Enlightenment version of *progress* envisions Western science as the primary engine of innovation and the means for achieving change that will lead to improvements in the viability and status of individuals. *National* and *international development* are particular types of progress: efforts to achieve more rapid realization of the Western Enlightenment-inspired notions of progress through planned and intentional action. The *international development field* comprises all national and international organizations, governmental and nongovernmental, mainly nonprofit but some for-profit, whose stated purpose is to promote national and international development or to support other organizations that are so engaged. As in all organizational fields, these organizations and their staffs have a mandate to promote a specific outcome and therefore conceive of themselves as actors or agents and value positive action over contemplation or study. Because of the number of entities able to act upon or be acted upon in the international development field, the organizations in this field are defined as a system of interdependent activities linking shifting coalitions of participants. Moreover, these systems are embedded in and dependent upon continuing exchanges with and constituted by the organizational environments in which they operate. For each organization identified, therefore, I provide a founding date (e.g., f. 1948) as a reminder that organizations are likely to carry in their procedures and staff some remnants of the era in which they were formed. In other words, none of these organizations operate independently of their organizational environment, both past and present.

Government organizations play particularly important legitimating and funding roles, and they tend to be organized along *bureaucratic* lines, with approved processes for carrying out specific activities assigned to specific bureaucratic positions. This introduces one of the central paradoxes of the field. International development professionals like to think of their work as mainly driven by *technical/efficiency* concerns, able to respond flexibly as countries and innovations vary. However, simply by the passage of time, many international development organizations have developed bureaucratic tendencies that resist innovation and variation.

International development aid represents transfers of technical assistance (usually in the form of experts), commodities, cash, and training from governments and nongovernmental organizations (NGOs) in industrialized countries to less industrialized countries with the stated aim of promoting national socioeconomic development. Whether the "aid" achieves this aim in specific cases or even most cases is, of course, arguable. International development aid is a subset of *foreign aid*, which also includes *security aid* to build military allies and *humanitarian aid*, aimed at relieving human suffering, whatever its source, ideally without regard for politics. Since the end of reconstruction after World War II, nation-states that did not participate in the Western Enlightenment have been the principal targets of most development aid. Over time, many of the experts and administrators who spend a substantial portion of their careers working in and for international development organizations see themselves as *development professionals* and exercise some jurisdiction (Abbott, 1988) over the ways development is defined and pursued, somewhat independent of donor and recipient nation-states. The terms *practitioner* and *professional* are used interchangeably throughout. Given the problematic nature of development, countries that tend to be recipients of development are referred to as *Third World countries*, *less-industrialized countries*, and *countries in the global South*.

An *institution,* consistent with the discussion above, is a social order or pattern that has attained a certain stable state that requires no active effort to maintain (Jepperson, 1991), but demands substantial, often collective action to change (DiMaggio, 1988). In popular usage, marriage, higher education, and the Internal Revenue Service are often referred to as institutions, and indeed they are somewhat consistent with this definition. In neo-institutionalist terms, the blueprints, scripts, and identities produced and carried by the organizations and professionals in the international development field generate the pressure to create and pursue global goals. Development professionals have developed step-by-step "best practices," or *blueprints,* for implementing specific activities in their pursuit of international development. The blueprint for promoting global goals, for example, includes global conferences, publications of scientific background papers, regional forums, national frameworks for action, and global monitoring reports, to name a few. Among the *scripts* that development professionals carry forward most forcefully are imperatives to rationalize, to quantify, to measure, and to standardize development activities in order to establish a rational basis for policy decisionmaking. The chief mechanisms professionals use to advance these scripts are discourse and funding. The degree to which these professionals are actors who are captains of their fate or are socialized to enact identities remains open to debate.

Finally, professionals often develop an insider language, including a dizzying array of acronyms, to refer to the organizations, practices, and concepts peculiar to their field. Those who aspire to study or work in any field must learn its insider language. For the sake of the more general reader, with the first mention of the full name of each organization or activity, I provide the founding date, the common acronym, and, as necessary, a two- or three-word abbreviated name. For example, I refer to the Pak-SEATO Cholera Research Laboratory (1961–1972, PS-CRL, the Cholera Lab) in Chapter 4 and to its successor, the International Center for Diarrheal Disease Research, Bangladesh (f. 1973, ICDDR,B, the Diarrhea Center) in Chapters 5 and 6. Note that many who are familiar with those organizations will know the acronym but may not recognize the two-word, abbreviated organizational name used in this book.

CONCLUSIONS

This book explores some of the ways innovations have shaped the pursuit of global goals in health and education in the last 30 years. To accomplish this, the analysis digs deeply into the history of two of the innovations that were expected to speed the realization of Health for All and Education for All. This analysis is particularly timely, as the international community is in the process of defining new global goals for the post-2015 era. Both HFA and EFA were originally defined in expansive terms, encompassing all stages of the life span. A few years after their initial declaration, however, both HFA and EFA were narrowed to focus on children, in the Child Survival and Universal Primary Education initiatives, respectively. The translation of both initiatives into Millennium Development Goals narrowed global health and education goals yet further. Failure to clearly achieve those narrower goals in more than 3 decades for HFA and 2 decades for EFA has, curiously, only increased pressure to return to the more expansive goals of both.

This book aims to inform and provoke scholars, students, and practitioners of international development and education to think more deeply about both the cultural and scientific underpinnings of education and international development. As such, it will probably have too little analysis for scholars, too much detail for students, and too much theory for practitioners. This is not a story that can be summarized in a graph or two; rather, the data are diverse and scattered through the weeds. The critique of many core principles of this sector within that field does not aim to undermine them, but rather to identify some of the lesser-known mechanisms and levers that influence the field. For those professionals in international development agencies who remain committed, against long odds, to realizing global education goals, this analysis may help identify some ways to put these mechanisms and levers to use. For scholars of international organizations and graduate students who aspire to join either the practitioners or the scholars in this field, this analysis identifies some new activities and some new areas for further research, respectively, that will welcome new talent.

CHAPTER 2

Imagining

From Universal Rights to Universal Goals

Mr. President, honorable delegates, ladies and gentlemen, *ce n'est pas des lois qu'il faut parler, c'est des moeurs.* It is not of laws that we should speak; it is of morals. The French social philosopher Montesquieu expressed sentiments to that effect nearly 250 years ago. . . . The quest for morality in human affairs laid the spiritual foundation . . . [that was the impetus] for social revolutions aimed at political equity . . . and today . . . at health equity. For without vision inspired by morality, the goal of health for all by the year 2000 could never have been conceived [and] . . . will never be attained.

—"World Health—2000 and Beyond,"
Halfdan Mahler, director-general, World Health Organization,
address to the World Health Assembly
(World Health Organization, 1988, p. 91)

The Millennium Development Goals (MDGs, f. 2000) are the latest in a series of efforts by international organizations to promote material and social progress, that is, socioeconomic development, as a human right on a global scale in the post-World War II period. Some international development professionals like Mahler, above, couch these efforts in terms of a secular morality explicitly linked to the Western Enlightenment, for whom Montesquieu (1689–1755) was an exemplary spokesperson. Others frame these goals as simply rational self-interest, a matter of national security for those who believe that deprivation leads to conflict, or a source of greater profit for those who calculate that increased prosperity leads to increased trade. This chapter aims to demonstrate the extent to which the global Health for All (HFA) initiative, referred to above by Mahler, served as a blueprint for the later global Education for All (EFA) initiative. Both were propelled by similarly mixed motives. Additionally, the chapter argues that many issues health and education experts may assume are unique to their respective sectors are, in fact, common to both when it comes to global initiatives.

CONSTRUCTING EDUCATION AND HEALTH AS HUMAN RIGHTS

Prior to World War II, socioeconomic development was something each nation-state had sole responsibility to promote—or not—within the borders of its country or empire. In the last half of the 20th century, however, a series of factors combined to erode that autonomy. Four are of particular interest here: the promulgation of a Universal Declaration of Human Rights; the decolonization of Africa and Asia; optimism spurred by the Marshall Plan that raising countries (mainly former colonies) out of extreme poverty would be possible within a decade or two; and the Cold War.

First, in 1948, the new United Nations issued the Universal Declaration of Human Rights, a document that framed social and economic progress in terms of human rights to a degree not found in prior international documents. According to the declaration, every living human being has rights, among other things, to

- social security, which is to be supported through national and international cooperation (Article 22);
- "a standard of living adequate for the health and well-being of himself [sic] and of his family, including food, clothing, housing, and medical care and necessary social services," as well as support and security in the event of unemployment, "sickness, disability, widowhood, old age, or other lack of livelihood beyond his control" (Article 25); and
- free, compulsory education, at least in the elementary and fundamental stages (Article 26).

This nonbinding declaration was translated into two binding international covenants in 1966 and ratified by most countries by 1976. The Covenant on Civil and Political Rights (the CPR Covenant) was championed by the capitalist West, principally the United States,[1] and makes no statements about health or education. The Covenant on Economic, Social, and Cultural Rights (the ESCR Covenant), in contrast, was championed by the Second World.[2] Article 12 of the ESCR Covenant, in 181 words, guarantees "the right of everyone to the enjoyment of the highest attainable standard of physical and mental health." Article 13, in twice as many words, guarantees the right of everyone to education that shall

- be directed to the full development of the human personality and the sense of its dignity;
- strengthen the respect for human rights and fundamental freedoms;

- enable all persons to participate effectively in a free society, promote understanding, tolerance, and friendship among all nations and all racial, ethnic, or religious groups, and further the activities of the United Nations for the maintenance of peace.

In these articles, the goals of education are much broader than those of health, guaranteeing "the full development of the human personality" and "enabling all persons to participate effectively in a free society."

Second, the ESCR Covenant created an international discourse around the right of each person to improve his or her material standard of living and to seek international aid to achieve it. For example, Part II, Article 11 states:

> The States Parties to the present Covenant recognize the right of everyone to an adequate standard of living . . . and *to continuous improvements* of living conditions. *The States Parties will take appropriate steps to ensure the realization of this right,* recognizing to this effect the essential importance of *international cooperation* based on free consent. [emphasis added]

This line of reasoning picked up momentum in the post–World War II period as dozens of former colonies gained independence and promptly ratified both covenants in principle. In many of these cases, national accession to universal rights to health and education was essentially aspirational. Only two countries made declarations to temper Article 12 (Health), whereas 14 made declarations in association with the more complex Article 13 (Education).

For example, Bangladesh (f. 1971) acceded to the ESCR Covenant in 1998, but also declared that it would implement all its provisions "in a progressive manner, in keeping with the existing economic conditions and the development plans of the country."[3] At the time, both Germany and Finland protested that these "declarations" constituted less than full acceptance of the ESCR Covenant. By 1998 "progressive realization" of global human rights standards, particularly for those countries with the lowest standards of living, was a well-established script, signaling limited government budgets and implementation capacity.

Third, the rapid success of the Marshall Plan in reconstructing Europe after World War II led some in Western countries to imagine that socioeconomic development consistent with the two human rights covenants could be achieved in less industrialized countries equally swiftly. The United Nations declared the 1960s *the* Development Decade, but the Second Development Decade soon followed in the 1970s. In 1974, the World Health Organization (f. 1948, WHO) and the United Nations Educational, Scientific and

Cultural Organization (f. 1946, UNESCO) launched, respectively, their first Universal Child Immunization and Universal Primary Education initiatives, both to be achieved by 1990. In 1980, at the beginning of the Third United Nations Development Decade, U.N. General Assembly Resolution 35/56 declared, among other goals, "infant mortality rates should reach 50 per 1,000 live births, as a maximum, by the year 2000" [December 5, para 48]. To this end, "Countries will establish an adequate and comprehensive system of primary health care as an integral part of a general health system." The General Assembly also declared support for "the provision of education on the broadest possible scale, the eradication or considerable reduction of illiteracy, and the closest possible realization of universal primary education [would be achieved] by the year 2010."

Fourth, the achievement of these goals presumed a higher level of co-operation and coordination among donor countries than has materialized. From 1946 to 1991, countries that had been World War II allies split into two factions—the capitalist or mixed economies of the First World and the communist Second World—and conducted what came to be known as the Cold War. Although driven by realistic concerns with power and security, the Cold War created a stream of funding that enabled international development to emerge as a field. First and Second World countries, most located in the global North, fought proxy wars largely in the global South. Communists and capitalists alike competed for influence—and sometimes military bases—in the newly independent and less industrialized countries with offers of both military and development aid. From the perspective of the global North, the South was rich in natural resources critical to the industrial growth of both Cold War antagonists, and the growing and modernizing populations of the global South constituted potential markets for Northern goods.

UNESCO became a battleground for the First and Second Worlds; the Soviets reluctantly ratified the CPR Covenant and the Americans refused to ratify the ESCR Covenant. In consequence, even though UNESCO, and later the United Nations Commission on Trade and Development (f. 1964, UNCTAD) and the United Nations Development Programme (f. 1966, UNDP), had been designed to direct and coordinate global development efforts, the largest First World countries would not channel the majority of their development assistance through them. Instead, in the 1960s, the more prosperous countries in the global North created bilateral development assistance organizations of their own devising, such as the U.S. Agency for International Development (USAID) and the British Overseas Development Agency (ODA), now the Department for International Development (DfID). In addition to giving donor countries greater control over how their resources were used, this arrangement made explicit to recipient countries to which side in the Cold War they were beholden. The United States maintained better working relations with the World Bank, the UNDP, and UNICEF. In recognition of the United States' large contribution to these organizations, the U.S. vote was calibrated to its contributions. The Soviet Union tended to have more influence in UNESCO, WHO, and the International Labor Organization (ILO).

DOES TALK MATTER?

In the U.N. General Assembly, the World Health Assembly, and the UNES-CO General Conference, each country has one vote. Third World countries, by banding together, can get some of their concerns on the agenda of these assemblies, even if they can't always get the donor countries to provide funds to address those concerns. Similarly, U.N. agencies, with budgets a small fraction of what their mandates require, nonetheless have the power to convene global meetings in their areas of specialization, independent of whether funds can be found to implement the recommendations those conferences and studies produce. As a result, U.N. agencies, the meetings they convene, and the studies they commission have sometimes been characterized as "talk shops," with little impact on the well-being of the world's poor. However, in a world where rationality is highly valued and where communication is making it easier for world culture to encroach on local approaches, talk may take on a life of its own (Chabbott, 2003).

For example, in 1972 Third World members succeeded in getting the U.N. General Assembly to declare a New International Economic Order (NIEO, or the New Order) that would obligate large income transfers from the First World to the Third. The New Order framed these transfers in part as reparation for past colonial injustices and in part as self-interest on the part of the global North in establishing steady trade flows with growing markets in a more prosperous global South. Nonetheless, several of the largest donors to development did not, literally, buy into the New Order. Instead, these donors framed the disappointing results of the First Development Decade as the result of too much emphasis on industrial development—the presumed primary engine of growth up to that time—and large-scale agriculture. Both of these emphases tended to benefit the owners of factories and larger farms—in short, elites. In the 1970s, these donors, rather, pledged to focus more resources on "basic human needs" and, subsequently, used the term "basic" to signal their intention to target program activities to non-elites. UNICEF, more dependent on the United States than most multilaterals and therefore always headed by a U.S. citizen, attempted to stake out a middle ground, framing its work in terms of a basic services approach.

Both the failure of the First Development Decade and talk throughout the Second Development Decade about the poor getting poorer motivated both humanitarians and realists in the First World to look for new mechanisms to channel development aid more directly to the poor rather than solely through their governments. The former looked to fulfill the idealism of the ESCR Covenant. The latter argued that education might raise the Third World out of poverty, thus addressing rising expectations and reducing the risk of violent overthrow of capitalists by the masses.

THE 1970s: HEALTH AND EDUCATION ON THE SAME TRACK

In the 1970s attention in the international development field shifted from industrialization and large-scale agriculture to human resources: health, population control, and education. This was the decade during which the concept of human capital (Schultz, 1961) came to the fore, emphasizing both health and education as key determinants of such capital. During this decade, the activities of nongovernmental organizations (NGOs), many at work in Third World countries since colonial times, provided proof that low-cost interventions could advance the quality of health and education in many impoverished communities.

Table 2.1 highlights parallels in the activities that promoted more action around universal rights to basic health care and education at the global level, beginning in the 1960s. Through most of the 1970s, efforts to expand access to primary health care and basic education in Third World countries received equal attention at the global level, but by the end of the decade, cooperation between two key agencies foundered on education while health surged ahead.

Getting to Health for All

During the 1950s and 1960s, WHO followed a single disease approach, experiencing heady success in eradicating smallpox, but also suffering notable setbacks, amplified by Cold War rivalries. Both technical and Cold War issues forced a change in approach in the 1970s. For example, a 1968 evaluation demanded by the Soviet delegate to the WHO's governing body, Dmitry Venediktov, concluded that efforts to "eradicate" malaria using DDT, largely funded by the United States, had failed. This same Venediktov later proposed that WHO undertake as its next major study "the scientific or rational principles upon which the development of a national public health system should be based" (Litsios, 2002). The delegate asserted that the problem of basic health services had been solved in the Soviet Union and

Table 2.1. Evolution of Global Goals for Health for All and Education for All

Sequence of Activities	Health	Education
International organizations form around Third World issues by sector	World Council of Churches—Christian Medical Commission (f. 1968)	International Institute for Educational Planning (f. 1963, IIEP)
Western experts identify sectoral crises in the Third World	*Health & the Developing World* (Bryant, 1969)	*World Educational Crisis* (Coombs, 1968)
International experts critique modern Western approach by sector	*Medical Nemesis* (Illich, 1976)	*Pedagogy of the Oppressed* (Freire, 1970) *Deschooling Society* (Illich, 1970)
International experts compile case studies of innovations in small-scale, community-based basic services delivery	*Health by the People* (Newell, 1975) *Alternative Approaches to Meeting Basic Health Needs* (Djukonovic & Mach, 1975)	*Attacking Rural Poverty: How Nonformal Education Can Help* (Coombs & Ahmed, 1974a) *Building New Education Strategies to Serve Rural Children and Youth* (Coombs & Ahmed, 1974b)
U.N. agencies organize global conference	WHO, UNICEF	UNESCO, UNICEF, World Bank, UNDP
Global declaration calls for comprehensive national plans of action	Health for All Alma-Ata, Kazakhstan (1978)	Education for All Jomtien, Thailand (1990)
Large funders focus on children and selective innovations	Child Survival (1981)	Universal Primary Education (1992)
Selective focus permits global goals	Reduce mortality rate for children under 5 years old by half by 2000	All children complete a full primary education by 2015 (Dakar Goal 6, 2000)

proposed an international conference in one of the Soviet republics to introduce the rest of the world to their successes (Venediktov, 1998). The delegate from the U.K., surprisingly for one coming from a First World country, supported this approach, saying that most of WHO's organizational studies to date "had been relatively sophisticated and perhaps were of interest only to the more developed countries," an approach that resonated equally well with both New Order and basic human needs proponents (Litsios, 2002).

Halfdan Mahler, who had recently been promoted to director-general, strongly opposed the top-down, medicalized direction in which the Soviets would have led WHO. Mahler's work in India in the 1950s had demonstrated to him that tuberculosis could be treated cheaply, at home, and that great gains in public health could be made with simple, low-cost innovations, outside of hospitals. With this conviction, Mahler wrote,

> [We went] with tears in our eyes to the Minister and we said, "Madame Minister, now that we have shown you this, you will have to close down all your tuberculosis hospitals because we need the money in order to do the ambulatory kind of treatment" and she looked at me and said, "You must be a crazy man, even an elephant would cry over your naïveté. How do you think I as a politician can close down the hospitals? You must be mad." (Litsios, 2002, p. 717)

In his first annual report for WHO, Mahler wrote that, as there are few models to

> demonstrate that primary health care can come out of the villages at a reasonable cost and in a matter that is technically acceptable, . . . [it is] an urgent task for WHO to seek a number of innovator countries that will be willing and able to set up such systems of primary health care and demonstrate their effectiveness. (Litsios, 2002, p. 718)

Thus Mahler ensured that a conference on a topic so close to his heart would not be captured entirely by formal, large-scale medicine. He found much international support for his position, including Ivan Illich's 1976 critique of modern medicine, *Medical Nemesis,* and a partnership with UNICEF, courtesy of Henry Labouisse, the low-key American executive director of UNICEF, someone well schooled in navigating the minefields of the Cold War.[4]

NGOs to the Rescue

By the 1970s, the main organizations engaged in community-based development approaches in the non-Communist Third World were small nongovernmental philanthropic or religious organizations. Of the latter organizations, Christian hospitals and schools were the principal providers of modern health care and formal education in many rural areas of sub-Saharan Africa for much of the 19th and the first half of the 20th century. However, as secularization rode into the last half of the 20th century on the coattails of modernization (Berger, 1999; Berger, Berger, & Kellner, 1973), the ranks of faith-based funders and future missionaries in the First World shrank. As former colonies became independent in the 1950s and 1960s, Third World church leaders transformed Christian missions into national churches and began a struggle to maintain the costly legacy of associated schools and hospitals. In response, the World Council of Churches created a Christian Medical Commission (f. 1968, CMC or the Commission) to help national churches in the Third World evaluate the role of approximately 1,200 missionary hospitals and to rethink how their work might be reengineered to provide better preventive care to more people (World Council of Churches, n.d.).

The Commission had only five full-time staff members, but it had member organizations in most Third World countries and heavy-hitting board members. The latter included John Bryant, the author of the seminal Rockefeller Foundation-supported report *Health and the Developing World* (1969), as well as Carl Taylor, who later founded the International Program at the Johns Hopkins University School of Public Health. Bryant and Taylor, both children of missionaries, were emblematic of a new generation of expatriates who emphasized the scientific, rather than the spiritual, nature of what Westerners might contribute to the Third World. At the same time, like Mahler and Illich, the commission and its board were concerned about the overmedicalization and dehumanization of primary health care delivery (Taylor & Bryant, 2008).

In its early years, the Commission identified and published case studies of health services provided by the services' members. These case studies tended to emphasize holistic approaches and prevention. Several directly linked poor health and nutrition to low income and argued that the most effective means of improving health was through improving agriculture or other productive sectors (Litsios, 2004). At the beginning of the 1970s, the Commission provided some of the few case studies that fit Mahler's call for "primary health care . . . [approaches or interventions] come out of the villages at a reasonable cost." As such, the Commission's work featured prominently in two volumes of case studies compiled to illustrate the feasibility of community-based health care to the World Health Assembly (Djukonovic & Mach, 1975; Newell, 1975).

The Health for All Conference

Venediktov argued that the small-scale undertakings of the type the Commission was producing and, of course, the Soviet Union's many larger cases needed more thorough discussion than WHO's annual meeting could afford. He proposed an International Conference on Primary Health Care, and in 1975 he offered WHO US$2 million, conditioned on convening in the Soviet Union. WHO and UNICEF together hosted the conference, and a quickly formed NGO Committee on Primary Health Care provided much conference preparation assistance over the next 3 years.[5]

Eventually, about 3,000 participants representing 134 member states, 67 international organizations, and dozens of NGOs attended a 3-day event in Alma-Ata (now known as Almaty), Kazakhstan. Despite the high profile of China's "barefoot doctors" in the case studies that informed the conference, Cold War tensions between the U.S.S.R. and China precluded China's participation in the conference (Cueto, 2004). The Declaration of Alma-Ata, proclaiming that "an acceptable level of health for all the people of the world by the year 2000 can be attained" (Article X), was carefully crafted and vetted in advance of the conference, so its acceptance by the gathered delegates was assured. Thirty years after the conference, Mahler recalled,

> It was almost a spiritual atmosphere, not in the religious sense, but in the sense that people wanted to accomplish something great. . . . At the end of the conference, a young African woman physician in beautiful African garb read out the Declaration of Alma-Ata. Lots of people had tears in their eyes. . . . There was a kind of jubilation immediately afterwards. (World Health Organization, 2008a, pp. 747–748)

The declaration itself identified seven essential components of a comprehensive approach to primary health care.[6] No diseases were highlighted for special attention, no targets set for the achievement of discrete campaigns, no particular groups identified as higher priority, and each country was left to develop a national plan as it saw fit.

Education Rises

In the education sector, all of UNESCO's main programs—fundamental literacy in the 1950s, functional literacy in the 1960s, a half-dozen goal-setting regional conferences for ministers of education in the 1950s and 1960s, and adult literacy campaigns in dozens of countries—were drastically underfunded and yielded predictably disappointing results (Jones, 1990). UNESCO's devolution into a battleground for the Cold War and later the New Order resulted in the loss of much of its funding from the First World.[7] Therefore, despite UNESCO's mandate in the education sector, many of the conferences and meetings that eventually led to EFA took place in other venues.

Some of the early activities that laid the groundwork for EFA preceded early activities for HFA. As shown in Table 2.1, before Illich published his critique of modern medicine, he more famously wrote a critique of modern schooling, *Deschooling Society* (1970), the same year Paolo Freire published *Pedagogy of the Oppressed* (1970), later followed by Martin Carnoy's *Education as Cultural Imperialism* (1974). Each of these books, in different ways, challenged the notion that modern, conventional, formal schooling, as organized in the First, Second, and Third Worlds in the 20th century, could achieve the human rights described in the ESCR Covenant. Their radical tone did not resonate well with First World donors or the major philanthropic foundations that funded much public policy-relevant research in the United States in the 20th century. Nonetheless, at the same time that a Rockefeller Foundation-supported report was detailing the desperate state of public health in the Third World (Bryant, 1969), a U.S. government-supported study, *The World Educational Crisis,* (Coombs, 1968) sketched an equally desperate picture in education:

> The crisis examined here . . . has been brought on by the failure of educational systems to transform themselves rapidly enough to match the needs of a swiftly changing environment. The crisis can be expected to deepen as education systems become more brutally squeezed between their rising unit costs and a slowdown in the rate of growth of financial resources. The only way out of the predicament, in the author's view, is through far-reaching educational *innovations*. . . . Merely to keep making the old educational system larger, he holds, will invite disaster. (jacket copy, emphasis added)

Coombs's study was the background paper for a U.S.-sponsored international conference on the same subject held in Williamsburg, Virginia, in October 1967. This meeting marked the beginning of a specialization in education within the international development field.

The Williamsburg conference was followed by high-level meetings for the heads of the World Bank, UNICEF, UNESCO, and most bilateral aid organizations in 1972 and 1973 at the Rockefeller Foundation Conference Center in Bellagio, Italy. Out of the series of education meetings in Bellagio came several new projects and networks, including the International Education and Reporting Service (f. 1974, IERS, the Reporting Service), which helped to establish a network of regional education innovation centers[8] and published the first case study series of innovations in education.[9] Mirroring Alma-Ata's focus on basic services delivery in 1978, the Reporting Service issued two volumes of case studies, together totaling more than 450 pages (UNESCO-UNICEF Cooperative Programme, 1978) on basic education services for children. Meanwhile, with funding from UNICEF and the World Bank, Coombs highlighted what he and many others perceived to be the solution to that crisis: community-based nonformal education for children and adults provided by both government and NGOs (Ahmed & Coombs, 1975; Coombs & Ahmed, 1974a, 1974b; Coombs, Ahmed, & Prosser, 1973).

Thus in the mid-1970s, health and education as sectors in international development had secured equal amounts of attention on the international development stage, from both the First and Second Worlds, focusing on "basic health services" and "basic education" for the Third World, consistent with the larger discourse on basic human needs. Both approaches depended upon NGOs to produce quicker, simpler approaches that international development organizations expected to scale-up to help meet ambitious global targets. However, while the health conference that would launch Health for All was just around the corner, a conference to launch EFA would be delayed for a dozen years.

THE 1980s: HEALTH AND EDUCATION DIVERGE

In 1980, a few months after he was appointed to be executive director of UNICEF, James P. Grant made a low-profile trip to Paris to meet with Amadou-Mahtar M'Bow, UNESCO's director-general, hoping to make education UNICEF's first priority for the next 10 years. The trip was a failure; M'Bow did not want to share leadership in education with any other agency. Moreover, M'Bow's determination to make UNESCO a champion of the New Order and his management style contributed to the United States, the United Kingdom, and Singapore withdrawing from UNESCO a few years later, financially crippling the organization. The notion of a partnership in education between UNICEF and UNESCO was not broached again until 1988, after Federico Mayor succeeded M'Bow at UNESCO and began the process of trying to woo the United States and the United Kingdom back into UNESCO. In the meantime, Grant returned to New York and continued his predecessor's focus on health, if in a very different way than either Mahler or Labouisse had envisioned.

Exploring the Selective Track

From its earliest days, many criticized the health services delivery and later the primary health care approaches for being too broad and, by extension, too costly. The bottom-up approach did not appeal to many officials in ministries of education who had risen through the ranks using top-down planning and had little contact with small-scale humanitarian community-based activities in rural areas. On the other hand, those not committed to or lacking experience with central planning were reluctant to believe that the public sector in a Third World country would be able to accomplish something many First World countries, such as the United States, had not.[10] Feasibility concerns aside, key international donors, such as the United States, were not willing to give less industrialized countries blank checks to build complete health systems, whether from the top down or from the bottom up.

In April 1979, less than a year after Alma-Ata and a year before Grant was appointed to UNICEF, a paper presented at Rockefeller's Bellagio Center at a meeting on Health and Population in Developing Countries made a case for "Selective Primary Health Care" (Walsh & Warren, 1979). In light of incomplete funding for all HFA components, the authors proposed a systematic process for setting priorities for HFA, based on available statistics. First, identify the infectious diseases that were causing the most harm to the most people. Then, rank those diseases by feasibility of control based on the effectiveness of the technology for treatment and the cost of treatment. This process produced a list of six high-priority diseases: diarrheal diseases, measles, malaria, whooping cough, schistosomiasis, and neonatal tetanus. Rebuttals to the paper appearing in medical journals later that year pointed out that this method came close to recommending a one-size-fits-all approach to public health; that it relied on questionable data; and, in addition, that it overlooked variations in the different sorts of capacity necessary to deliver different high-priority interventions (Berman, 1982; Gish, 1982; Lipkin, 1982).

Child Survival as a Selective Track

In 1982 Grant heard a young doctor give a compelling speech on "How the Other Half Dies" (Rohde, 1982). Using widely available statistics, Jon Rohde argued that each year about 14 million deaths of children under 5 years old in the developing world were "unnecessary." Most of these children were dying from five or six common illnesses—measles, tetanus, whooping cough, pneumonia, and diarrheal disease—that were cheaply and easily treatable. Rohde challenged his audience to build a bridge between "what science knew and what people needed" (Adamson, 2001, p. 21). He also argued that the main obstacle was not scientific but political: getting political leaders to allocate the money and to support effective programs.

This notion provided Grant with the rationale for a selective approach to promoting child health that he hoped might achieve the scope and impact of the Green Revolution in agriculture, which he had witnessed in India and Turkey in the 1960s. In 1982, in his third annual *State of the World's Children* report, Grant announced that UNICEF would launch a Child Survival and Development Revolution to halve the mortality rate for children under 5 years old (the under-5 mortality rate, U5MR) by the year 2000. The Child Survival strategy, he said, would be based on four interventions: growth monitoring, oral rehydration therapy for diarrheal diseases, breast-feeding, and immunizations for several childhood diseases, soon referred to collectively as GOBI.[11] These interventions addressed two of the three main killers of children under 5: vaccine-preventable diseases and diarrheal diseases.[12] As noted earlier in this chapter, the international community had already committed itself to universal child vaccination by 1990, and new ways to keep vaccines cold in the field had recently increased the possibilities for getting them to remote areas (Nyi Nyi, 2001). The efficacy and cost-effectiveness of oral rehydration therapy and immunizations had been scientifically established with randomized, controlled trials, or at least large-scale statistically validated surveys. All four were low-cost and could benefit from recent advances in communications; all except immunization involved behavior change rather than costly, imported medicine.

Those close to Grant during this period argue that he did not see GOBI as the final answer to Health for All but as "low-hanging fruit" that could give the world a taste for success in public health. He argued that success would generate political commitment and financial resources to build more comprehensive programs of primary health care and rural development, country by country (Adamson, 2001; Nyi Nyi, 2001). To many, the discrete, stand-alone components of GOBI, however, looked suspiciously like WHO's repudiated top-down, single-disease campaigns for malaria and yaws; none of the components built sustainable primary health care systems. Mahler, among others, saw this as a threat to the united front that health experts needed to maintain to get donor and recipient countries to do the hard work of building comprehensive primary health systems, tailored to each country, from the bottom up. Many questioned the quality of life for children who simply "survived" to age 5 and faced a life without access to a primary health care system.

Cases Help Build the Case for Child Survival

Attempting to bridge the gap between HFA and Child Survival, Rohde and public health professor David Morley assembled 18 case studies to illustrate

> that effective and affordable health technologies do exist for dealing with the major health problems of the South. The main obstacles to the implementation of these technologies, however, are not technical but political and organizational. (Morley, Rohde, & Williams, 1983, p. x)

Many of these cases had not managed to lay down baseline data, and the medical effectiveness of their implementation methods could not be established in quantitative terms. The most successful cases were complex, including activities formally outside the health sector, such as income generation and agriculture. None of these cases offered any hope of quick, predictable results, and the idea of building political commitment did not appeal to many experts in international health, who continued to imagine development as a process mainly driven by universal technologies and quantitative evidence.

Nonetheless, in 1984 the heads of the Rockefeller Foundation, the World Bank, USAID, WHO, and UNDP attending a conference at the Bellagio Conference Center joined UNICEF in forming a Task Force on Child Survival. Three years into the Child Survival initiative, in May 1985, UNICEF sponsored a conference to discuss progress to date, alternative strategies, and future directions (Cash, Keusch, & Lamstain, 1987). At the conference Grant articulated why the selected interventions were so compelling: they could be described in terms simple enough that parents could understand and act; they were (relatively) inexpensive to put into operation (no more than $10 per child); they were universal in relevance and synergistic in their relationships; and, finally, they were not dependent on profound changes in values or priorities. "Drastically improved child health and survival is thereby made realistic by shifting its operational center of gravity from health institutions to the family itself" (Cash, Keusch, & Lamstain, 1987, p. ix). For some, however, it looked like these interventions allowed governments to abdicate earlier commitments to the ESCR Covenant and HFA.

Just 4 months later, the Rockefeller Foundation convened a meeting on "Good Health at Low Cost" to address "the interest of some of us in developing a global strategy for achieving 'Health for All' by targeting for action an essential short list of diseases" (Rockefeller Foundation, 1985, p. 5). The announcement continued: "A guarantee of a long life to nearly everyone cannot wait the attainment of global affluence. It now appears that it does not have to. There is an available model" (p. 7).

At the meeting, William B. Greenough III, the director of the research center that had developed one of the GOBI interventions, oral rehydration therapy, presented the only paper focused entirely on selective interventions (Greenough, 1985). He identified seven interventions that did not require physicians to deliver them, beginning with soap—which, he said, had the potential to do more to reduce mortality than more costly water and sanitation projects—then ORT, breast-feeding, indigenous medicine, nutrition, family planning, and vaccines. He concluded,

> I have pointed to vast chasms of ignorance because of failure to do what is necessary—rigorous field tests of health measures that are to be widely applied. Despite this, the four countries under review, by tapping their own traditions and empiric wisdom, have shown us *what can be accomplished without the rigorous process of science.* (p. 218, emphasis added)

Greenough reminded the audience that simple, low-cost interventions that can be administered by nonprofessionals outside formal medical establishments could not be copyrighted and, in the process, undercut physicians, hospitals, and drug company profits and provoked their resistance. Finally, he emphasized the importance of nonexperimental research approaches in epidemiology and sociology. As an example, he reported, "Under conditions of famine in Bangladesh, survival of children of educated mothers was six times greater than that of their neighbors with equal resources" (Greenough, 1985, p. 216). Yet, he said, little work had been done to objectively define what educated mothers do to accomplish this.

Each of the case studies presented at the meeting began with an analysis of statistical indicators. Indicators were also critical for the "selling" of Child Survival to both politicians and donors.

The Role of Indicators

HFA had chosen infant mortality as one of its two goal indicators, but for the Child Survival initiative, Grant chose the U5MR. UNICEF's mandate clearly covered more than just infants, he reasoned, and the U5MR was a larger, more dramatic number, which made fundraising and social mobilization easier. However, in many of the countries with the highest levels of child mortality, few births or deaths, at any age, were officially reported.[13] For several years, therefore, lacking these vital statistics, UNICEF inferred the U5MR from an amalgamation of sources.

Although the estimates of U5MR had and, in some places, still have large margins of error, Grant insisted on using them as a communications tool. In sharp contrast with his low-key predecessors at UNICEF, he crisscrossed the globe with a string of celebrity UNICEF ambassadors, reasoning with, cajoling, and vexing Third World leaders into supporting immunization drives and ORT use. He was, both friends and detractors say, shameless in his efforts to persuade donor and recipient countries to take action immediately; he carried little bottles of chemicals in his pockets to test the salt at state dinners to verify that commitments to iodize salt had been met. He made dictators and saints alike vaccinate children on television, in order to demonstrate its safety and publicly endorse whatever combination of short-listed GOBI-FFF interventions the leaders had been persuaded to endorse (Adamson, 2001). "Who can say 'no' to children?" he demanded. A UNICEF regional director describes Grant's drill as his team swept into UNICEF country offices for a day or two:

> He would list in a small notebook in his shirt pocket some five points that he expected to raise. [He demanded from] the [UNICEF country] representative . . .

key information—how many children under 5 die per day in that country? This information would be transformed into the equivalent number of Boeing 757s filled to capacity crashing each day. . . . What are the immunizations rates this year compared to last year? How many mothers use oral rehydration salts? . . . What proportion of children has growth cards? Armed with this information, he would start his fishing expedition [with the prime minister or president]. . . . Casting out the first line of conversation, he would assess whether the president was going to bite. If the latter showed only mild, courteous interest, out would come the next line, with the lure in the form of his famous visual aids. There was the tried and true packet of oral rehydration salts, or the restaurant match-book with child survival messages on the igniting side. If this line of conversation sparked an interest . . . he would firm up the line and gradually reel in the big fish. . . .

What the president and his protocol officer assumed would be only a half-hour courtesy visit would soon turn into an hour-long working session. The president would at some point promise to devote quarterly cabinet meetings to reviewing progress in child immunization. Or the prime minister would agree to speak with five other especially influential presidents and prime ministers at the next Organization for African Unity meeting to ensure the appropriate wording on oral rehydration use would go into their final resolutions. (Racelis, 2001, p. 132)

On the plane leaving these countries, Grant would prepare a memorandum of understanding covering the agreements he had extracted and promptly dispatch it to the prime minister or president, to be followed up regularly by the UNICEF country director and by Grant himself, as needed (personal communication, James P. Grant, August 1994).

In the face of this public relations/social mobilization blitz, nongovernmental and governmental organizations alike lined up to fund specific interventions, such as polio vaccination (Rotary), oral rehydration (Boy Scouts), iodized salt (Kiwanis), vitamin A (Helen Keller International), and family planning and oral rehydration[14] (USAID). UNICEF field offices in Third World countries were stretched to the limits of their implementation capacity. Other more holistic health strategies, perhaps years in the making, were laid aside. In conflict areas, UNICEF persuaded belligerents to lay down their arms long enough for children to be vaccinated, and UNICEF staff marched across the temporarily suspended battle lines carrying their iceboxes full of vaccines. It was, indeed, a moralizing crusade, calling for unique, heroic efforts, intended to take a chunk out of the U5MR while, presumably, governments were constructing more solid foundations for a long-term primary health care system.

THE 1990s: EDUCATION COMES IN FROM THE COLD

The third meeting of the Task Force on Child Survival, convened in March 1988 in Talloires, France, issued the Declaration of Talloires, citing as progress:

- more than 50% of infants in developing countries had been vaccinated, preventing some 200,000 children annually from being paralyzed by polio or dying from a preventable disease;
- lifesaving fluids were now available for 60% of the developing world's population, preventing as many as 1 million deaths annually from diarrhea;
- initiatives to control respiratory infections could prevent many of the 3 million childhood deaths annually.

A bit heady with progress to date, the declaration also reported progress on diseases not initially included in GOBI, such as respiratory infections. Further, it recommended that countries commit themselves to ambitious new goals for the year 2000, such as the global eradication of polio; the virtual elimination of neonatal tetanus deaths; and a 50% reduction in current maternal mortality rates. Finally, the declaration drew attention to the potential for enlarging upon these successes by improving the quality and coverage of educational services to raise female literacy rates to 80%.

Imagining Education Parallels to Child Survival and HFA

Education, particularly female education, had been connected to health since HFA's earliest days, but it was finally at Talloires that Grant reported being approached by a funder with resources for large-scale initiatives. The president of the World Bank, Barber Conable, asked Grant, "Isn't there something like this [Child Survival] that we could do for education?" Grant considered this a vindication of his strategy. Successes in selective health interventions indeed appeared to be leading to more support for broader initiatives beyond Child Survival, even beyond the health sector itself. About the same time, the new director-general of UNESCO, Federico Mayor, also approached Grant, looking for some way to launch an educational equivalent to the Child Survival Initiative, at least in part to restore UNESCO's legitimacy and to attract the United States and the United Kingdom back to the organization (personal communication, James P. Grant, August 1994).

Thus in 1988 a small group assembled in UNICEF's New York office, including senior staff from UNESCO's International Institute for Educational

Planning (f. 1963, IIEP, the Education Institute) and senior UNICEF staff, including Grant. In the course of the meeting Grant scandalized the Education Institute's staff when he demanded a number. He demanded them to tell him how much it would cost to make one child literate. He insisted that if a firm, "unconscionably" low price tag could be established, the money could be raised. No such price tag came out of that meeting or any other in the 15-month preparatory period for EFA. When UNICEF asked a meeting of major donor education advisors and staff in 1988 if a global conference might provide the spark necessary to start a basic education revolution, they did not reject the notion. Like their colleagues in health, many of the education experts were motivated by the prospect of establishing comprehensive, sustainable systems, that is, Education for All, but apparently they took what they could get.

Following the world conference blueprint used by HFA and by recent World Bank meetings, the conference preparation staff was drawn from the four sponsoring agencies: UNICEF, UNESCO, the World Bank, and UNDP. Like the one that prepared for Alma-Ata, this temporary group worked heroically but with far fewer people in less than half the time. To secure broader input into the conference documents—a declaration and framework for action—the EFA Secretariat scrambled to organize regional consultations with government and NGO representatives around hastily drafted declarations and frameworks. At their regional meeting, the African participants recalled earlier regional meetings organized by UNESCO that had pushed African states to declare ambitious targets—UPE in 1960, then in 1970—only to see funding promises evaporate and the Africans themselves blamed for a failure to meet the targets. They were fully aware that in most African countries, there were no baseline data upon which to make reliable estimates of growth in enrollments or completion. They declined to endorse any universal targets for EFA, and no one was prepared to calculate the cost of either conventional or innovative approaches.

Education for All in Practice

Greatly to Grant's disappointment, the EFA conference in Jomtien, Thailand, in March 1990 produced no global targets, nor did it uncover more than one or two potential fast-expanding, low-cost interventions, one of which features in Chapters 4 through 6 of this book. Nonetheless, like the HFA participants, many of the EFA participants recall the conference as one that called upon the highest ideals of development. In their recollection, as the Declaration of Education for All was read at the final ceremony, the stirring summons brought participants to their feet to accept it by acclamation, some with tears in their eyes that recalled the high emotions at the conclusion of the health conference at Alma-Ata. Coming down from the mountaintop of its closing ceremony, the EFA initiative faced many of the same issues HFA had at a similar stage, plus a few more. First, in its fullest sense, EFA implied comprehensive planning and flexible implementation capacity far beyond the experience of the countries that had the farthest to go to realize universal education:

> Three major sets of requirements [for moving EFA forward] were identified in [the conference] documents: developing a supportive policy context; mobilizing resources; and strengthening international solidarity. The discussions held at the Jomtien Conference suggested that a fourth requirement—building national technical capacity—should be added. (Windham, 1992, p. 1)

The capacity issue was not adequately addressed for the next 20 years. Instead, USAID and other donors provided grants to build technical capacity in education management information systems (EMIS) to track progress in schooling.

Second, although the preparation for EFA produced at least one major report on education indicators (Windham, 1988), the education community seemed to agree on just one thing: enrollment and completion rates, the only broadly available indicators of primary school progress, were not good proxies for learning and therefore did not constitute adequate measures of educational achievement. Simply completing five grades of primary school does not produce a decent quality of life and was no more acceptable to the international education community than U5MR had been to the health community. Moreover, an 80% vaccination rate could achieve virtual eradication of some diseases. Education, in contrast, was not contagious, and "all" would have to mean 100%. As in health, reaching the last 20%—in remote areas, among disadvantaged minorities, for children and adults with special needs, not to mention refugees—might be as expensive as reaching the other 80% combined. A joint UNESCO/UNICEF initiative, Monitoring Education for All Project: Focusing on Learning Achievement, finally began collecting baseline time series data on learning in 1992, but various configurations of donors would struggle with building consensus around an internationally comparable indicator for learning for the next 2 decades.

A price tag per learner remained elusive, because EFA was being talked about in terms of education systems—much like HFA's health systems—not in terms of discrete interventions. The dozen or so cost-effective and doable interventions for HFA had come to light after the 1978 conference. Consequently, it might not have troubled Grant and the other conveners of EFA that no such interventions appeared in the lead-up to the 1990 EFA conference. From a modernist perspective, if science had produced such interventions in one sector, why should it not do so in another? And if the science of education was lagging slightly behind the science of health, then might not the pressure created by the conference and its follow-up help to close that gap?

Finally, in looking for precedents for rapid national campaigns that had yielded relatively rapid results, UNICEF turned to, among other examples, literacy and primary education campaigns in Burma, Tanzania, and Nicaragua (Nyi Nyi, 1983; see also Ahmed, 1984; Le Boterf, 1984); case studies of primary education innovations found in compilations of education innovations established and maintained by UNESCO and UNICEF; and a handful of recent innovations (Anderson, 1992), most of them small-scale. These exemplars fostered the sense that the innovations necessary to attain EFA, or at least UPE, already existed and were ready to be modified and scaled up in new contexts. They sidestepped a pivotal issue: Who or what entity was going to adapt and deliver these existing innovations to the scores of distinctly difficult contexts where UPE was most needed?

Despite these uncertainties, the EFA Framework for Action encouraged national governments to develop National Plans of Action incorporating quantitative targets and goals for each "dimension" of education: early childhood, primary education, literacy, and vocational training for adults. Meanwhile the EFA High Level Group, like the Child Survival Task Force, met every 2 years to address key issues and report on progress, but no significant staff was appointed to assist with organizing meetings and to track and publicize progress, or lack of it. Thus it fell to host countries and individual development organizations to fund the meetings.

Education for All . . . Children

As had been the case with HFA, almost before the ink was dry on the EFA Declaration, major funders began backing away from a comprehensive approach. Few adult literacy campaigns since the end of World War II had succeeded in producing large numbers of people who could read and write fluently, let alone put those skills to use in such a way that generated more income or higher levels of well-being. Similarly, most youth vocational education programs were small-scale, organized in idiosyncratic ways by NGOs, and few had cost-effectiveness analyses even at that scale. Further, governments that had already made primary education compulsory and did not have the funds to cover it could not afford to fund noncompulsory early childhood education. Finally, to many development practitioners, higher education appeared too expensive and too elite-oriented, and benefited largely those who had already received more than their fair share of the national education budget.

UNICEF shored up the human rights case for UPE, already a global target since 1974, by including it in the Convention on the Rights of the Child (ratified 1990), thus legally binding all 191 signers to provide primary education. On the technical side, economists at the World Bank—the organization generating more highly legitimated quantitative education research than any other international development organization—had declared internal rates of return dramatically higher for primary than for any other level of education (Psacharopoulos & Woodhall, 1985). At EFA, World Bank President Barber Conable chaired the Roundtable on Primary Education and sponsored the first High Level Forum following the Jomtien conference on that same topic. The manuscript of a book prepared by two senior education experts at the World Bank, *Improving Primary Education in Developing Countries* (Lockheed & Verspoor, 1991), served as the basic background document for the roundtable and forum.

There was no effective resistance as the scope of EFA quickly narrowed. UNESCO had no economists to defend adult literacy or vocational training, nor significant funds of its own to invest in scientific research. Despite UNESCO's partnership with the three U.N. agencies most closely aligned with the United States, EFA did not immediately restore the United States or the United Kingdom, or their dues, to UNESCO. UNDP, with a relatively small budget compared to the World Bank's, had never been a major funder of education and did not become one after Jomtien. Immediately following the EFA conference, therefore, the two largest donors to education—the United States and the World Bank—determined that the majority of their funding would focus on access to formal primary schooling. UNICEF, with its mandate for children, its relatively small funding base, but its large bully pulpit, likewise focused on education for children.

After Grant's death in 1995, UNICEF's breakneck pace of the previous decade—spearheading Child Survival, ratifying the Convention on the Rights of the Child, launching Education for All—could not be sustained, and UNICEF refocused on a subset of UPE: girls' education. In the late 1990s, though the world came close to meeting the HFA targets, the growing HIV/AIDS epidemic diverted the funds necessary to close the deal, and some countries could not maintain their Child Survival achievements. EFA continued going through the motions of the world conference model throughout the 1990s, holding the Summit for the Nine Most Populous Countries in Delhi in 1993; the Mid-Decade Conference in Amman, Jordan, in 1996; several high-level forums; and the end-of-decade World Education Forum in Dakar, Senegal, in 2000. The results shared at Dakar were largely disappointing, and in response, time-bound, fixed, universal targets were established for 2010. Two years later, a subset of these targets relating to UPE and female education were rolled into the Millennium Development Goals, as described ahead in Chapter 7.

CONCLUSIONS

By the last half of the 20th century, notions of universal rights for all individuals and the necessity of international cooperation to realize them were formalized in the Universal Declaration of Human Rights and codified in two binding covenants. There remains much loose coupling between the rights to health care and education described in the ESCR Covenant and access to health care and schooling of good quality in much of the Third World. Much of this loose coupling has institutional roots.

Article 13 in the ESCR Covenant describes education as more central to achieving both material and social progress with equity than Article 12 does for health. At the same time, the covenant frames education as more complex and more countries placed reservations, including "progressive realization," on Article 13 than on Article 12. Many of these countries clearly lacked the funds and implementation capacity necessary to fulfill these commitments. Why did they ratify or accede at all? Did some countries regard signature of the covenant as normative, necessary to uphold their status as legitimate states, or were their leaders copying what other modern nation-states were doing? Did some hope to signal strong intentions to develop their countries to potential development donors? The United States, one of the largest donors to health, never ratified the ESCR Covenant, but the United Kingdom and France, both important education donors in former colonies, did. Did former colonies perceive education and health as really so central to development, or did they go along with the covenant in order to appeal to its "international cooperation" clauses? All of these reasons might help to explain why, beyond a shortage of development funds and implementation capacity, progress toward realization of rights to public health and, particularly, to education was slow in many countries.

The crises defined in health and education in the 1970s and 1980s consisted of gaps between universal rights articulated only a few decades earlier and conditions that had existed for millennia. Those gaps were social constructs that transformed age-old tragedies into crises demanding dramatic action in a decade or two. These crises gave WHO and UNESCO mandates to launch global initiatives. A multitude of low-income countries that looked to development aid to expand health and education service delivery had every institutional reason—resource dependence, coercive, normative, and/or mimetic—to adopt the universal goals associated with these initiatives. They did not, perhaps, anticipate the rationalization and pursuit of universal quantitative indicators at the national level. Several *generalizations* about *the role of world society in global initiatives emerge from this analysis:*

G2.1. Global initiatives that can be associated with prior formal commitments made at the global level, by many nation-states, gain legitimacy somewhat independent of the means to achieve them.

G2.2. Loose coupling between global goals and national/local actions will vary inversely with the degree of connection between a specific context and its participation in or contact with the Western Enlightenment.

G2.3. Over time, demand for nation-states to conform to international commitments to global goals will increase and the means for quantitatively tracking those commitments will multiply and become standardized.

HFA was among the pioneers of the global conference/declaration/goals blueprint. Twelve years later, based on HFA and other global conferences, EFA was able to convene in less than half the preparatory time needed by HFA. Leaders in HFA and EFA, specifically Mahler and Grant, drew inspiration from the earlier eradication of smallpox and the Green Revolution in agriculture. Both HFA and EFA implied comprehensive, costly, and lengthy reorganization of conventional health and education systems in many countries. In contrast, the selective version of HFA, Child Survival, and to a lesser extent Universal Primary Education for EFA, placed more emphasis on innovations. Over time, as the number of global initiatives increased, so, too, did the number of meetings associated with them. These meetings, such as those of the Task Force on Child Survival, provided new venues for leaders and professionals to interact and to theorize, share models, shore up identities, and tinker with scripts. The worldwide diffusion of theories offering to explain backwardness in specific sectors, such as Ivan Illich's *Medical Nemesis* (1976) and *Deschooling Society* (1970), as well as case studies of innovation that were published in connection with global conferences, provided a common basis for rationalizing appropriate responses. The notions of *blueprints, identities, and scripts* suggest several generalizations about the development of global initiatives over time:

G2.4. As more global initiatives are launched, a blueprint for global conferences/declarations/goals/global monitoring emerges, enabling new global initiatives to launch more quickly than older ones did.

G2.5. As the identity of modern, internationalist, humanitarian leader and of international development professional becomes established, champions for new global initiatives take less time to establish themselves.

G2.6. Successful scripts for promoting global initiatives will incorporate key world culture themes: equity (rights-based), material well-being (technical efficiency), and individualism (for all, humanitarian universalism).

Much of what occurred at the organizational level and below, however, is easily explained in terms of normal social science, with no special references to institutional factors. Although the participants clearly saw the role of the Cold War in the development of HFA, by all accounts, organizations and their leaders, not nation-states, shaped it, set it in motion, and sustained it. Halfdan Mahler and James Grant provided charismatic leadership for the conceptualization of HFA and Child Survival/EFA, respectively. All accounts suggest that they were convinced their role in WHO and UNICEF was to make something happen at the global level, running on a heady mix of moral conviction and a grueling work ethic, using science and mobilizing bureaucracies when it suited their causes, following and shoring up their work to ensure that it endured. Nonetheless, the funding limitations of WHO and UNESCO meant that the organizations with the formal mandates to operationalize the health and education provisions of the ESCR Covenant had to rely on others for funding. The available funders for HFA and EFA narrowed the scope of both. All of this suggests several unsurprising generalizations about *the role of organizations* in the process of launching and sustaining global initiatives:

O2.1. Funding organizations support at least some components of the initiative.
O2.2. Local organizations in some of the contexts with the farthest to go to meet the goals of the global initiative have:
  • piloted innovations relevant to some part of the initiative and established some as cost-effective, and
  • a mandate to act and are headed by one or more charismatic, competent innovators or leaders.
O2.3. Angel investors stand ready to support the early invention, adaptation, and piloting of new innovations.
O2.4. The initiative does not demand profound changes in culture and/or standard operating procedures in either implementing or funding organizations.

These generalizations could come from any textbook on organizational development. Similarly, much of what these cases reveal about the role of innovations in international initiatives echoes the literature on innovation (Adams & Chen, 1981; Rogers, 2003). Innovations are likely to be more useful in launching and sustaining global initiatives when they are:

I2.1. salient to initiative,

I2.2. simple,

I2.3. stand-alone,

I2.4. cheap to produce and deliver,

I2.5. in the public domain,

I2.6. do not demand unprecedented levels of sustained behavior change,

I2.7. amenable to social mobilization,

I2.8. produce results quickly,

I2.9. produce results that are dramatic, evident to the naked eye,

I2.10. validated with quick, cheap, universal outcome indicator(s), and

I2.11. authorized as universal by high science.

Finally, the HFA/CS and EFA/UPE cases highlight the importance of quantitative measurement in a world in which individuals, not groups, are the level at which equity and progress are measured. The construction of the U5MR was an important advance for the Child Survival initiative, something that resonated with politicians and bureaucrats, literate and illiterate, professionals and parents alike. Despite its technical sound, at least initially, its level was imputed, estimated, not empirically measured. Moreover, it represented a necessary and leading but not sufficient indicator on the road to a healthy life, in the same way that "children complete primary school" was a necessary and leading but not sufficient indicator for an education that enables a meaningful and productive life. Child Survival, however, could make a better humanitarian case than UPE could. Children have survived and many have thrived for millennia without formal education.

Grant was prescient about the importance of measurement. Between his meetings with global education experts, where he demanded an "unconscionably" low price tag to "make one child literate," and his whirlwind meetings with UNICEF staff in national offices, from whom he demanded devastating child health statistics, Grant clearly understood the levers that move modern politicians and funders. A late modern take on the Archimedean principle might be "Give me a *statistic* on which to stand, and I will move the Earth." Interventions that produce dramatic effects that are evident to the naked eye will be more useful than those whose impact is less observable. Likewise, low-cost measures that can quickly detect and summarize highly valued impact that is not visible to the naked eye will also be more valuable than other sorts of measures.

Child Survival promoters saw themselves in the vanguard of international development, hoping to turn success on "low-hanging fruit" interventions, such as child immunization or iodized salt, into broader support for primary health care. Indeed, the Task Force on Child Survival inspired many single-disease campaigns—malaria, guinea worm, AIDS—beyond GOBI in the decades after its founding, such that it evolved into the Task Force on Global Health, not the Task Force on Primary Health Care. Indeed, it was at a task force meeting that the possibility of EFA was first raised.

UPE, despite its uninspiring progress in the 1990s, got a new lease on life in the following decade. The Health for All and Child Survival documents are salted with references to the importance of female education; both the health and the family planning sectors helped to keep basic education, at least for girls, central to global discourse. Carol Bellamy, James Grant's successor at UNICEF, made girls' education the centerpiece of UNICEF's strategy. The Millennium Development Goal for gender equity is measured in terms of enrollments in education, and that has brought support for education goals from women's rights groups outside the education sector.

Nonetheless, for both Child Survival and UPE, progress to date, although much better than for HFA and EFA, falls far short of their least demanding targets, as shown in Table 2.2. At the same time, moral suasion, based on Western Enlightenment values, continues to generate support to pursue more expansive HFA and EFA goals, and Western science continues to generate cost-effective innovations for pursuing HFA, if not for EFA.

The health sector was not always so well equipped with science. In 1985, a senior Rockefeller Foundation official asserted that the Child Survival "revolution" was underachieving in comparison with its prototype, the Green Revolution in agriculture. He attributed this in part to the lack of international research centers "linked backward to fundamental research centers, mostly in the industrialized world, but increasingly also in the developing world" (Bell, 1987, p. 252).

Bell was in a position to make this comparison not just because the foundation had, over the previous 40 years, supported the development of a network of a dozen or so international agricultural research centers, but also because the Foundation had recently supported the development of one international health research center with similar forward and backward linkages. Two decades earlier, that research center, based in one of the poorest countries in the world, invented one of the four GOBI interventions, oral rehydration therapy. The next chapter explores what students of EFA might learn from the evolution of this center.

Table 2.2. Progress Toward Millennium Development Goals for Education and Health

GOAL 2: ACHIEVE UNIVERSAL PRIMARY EDUCATION						
Indicator	2015 Target		Start EFA 1990	1st decade 2000	2nd decade 2011	Achieve MDG by 2015?
Primary school completion rate*	Achieve 100%	World	80.5	82.4	90.6	No
		Developed regions	97.2	97.2	99.9	NA
		Sub-Saharan Africa	52.2	53.6	69.2	No
		South Asia, excluding India	56.3	61.2	68.2	No
		Least developed countries	40.8	45.8	63.7	No
GOAL 4: REDUCE CHILDHOOD MORTALITY						
Indicator	2015 Target		1st decade 1990	2nd decade 2000	3rd decade 2012	Achieve MDG by 2015?
Under-5 mortality rate (#/1,000)	Reduce 1990 rate by two-thirds	World	87	73	50	29: No
		Developed regions	15	10	6	5: Possible
		Sub-Saharan Africa	178	153	105	59: No
		South Asia, excluding India	119	87	58	40: No
		Least developed countries	171	136	95	57: No

*Total # new entrants to last grade of primary divided by the population of the theoretical age to enter that grade.

Source: mdgs.un.org/unsd/mdg/Host.aspx?Content=Data/Trends.htm

CHAPTER 3

Inventing

Carrot Soup, Magic Bullets, and Scientific Research

Gosh, maybe he's right.

> —Scientist's response when a country doctor told him his
> oral rehydration work was the most profound development
> in the treatment of cholera in the 20th century

Following the U.N. Millennium Summit in 2000, the Millennium Development Goals (MDGs) established for health and education reflected the incongruity between the two sectors described in the previous chapter. As shown in Table 3.1, the main targets for health were expressed in terms of outcomes, whereas the main target for education was expressed in terms of service delivery. Making the health targets congruent with the actual education target reduces them to "access to a health clinic," as shown in italics. Conversely, making the education target congruent with the health targets entails elevating it to actual levels of learning for specific groups, as shown in italics.[1]

The reason for the difference was simple: each of the MDGs was established to reflect reported progress in recent decades on existing indicators (Vandemoortele, 2011). Measurable progress on EFA in the 1990s was slow in many of the countries farthest from achieving it. Indeed, shortly after the MDGs were established, at least one analysis, based on 40 years of existing data, found the education MDG patently unattainable (Clemens, 2004).[2]

These results are consistent with arguments made at the 1990 Education for All (EFA) Conference that EFA could not be achieved with "business as usual," either in terms of funding or of existing education systems (Verspoor, 1993; World Conference on Education for All, 1990, Article 7).

The current chapter, discussing the inventing phase of an innovation, does not presume to resolve all the tension around which aspects of health and education research are commensurable and which are not. Rather, the analysis points to several areas for further consideration by those interested

Table 3.1. Targets for Millennium Development Goals

	Service Delivery	Outcome
Education	Achieve universal primary education.	*Reduce by two-thirds the number of children who cannot read fluently at age 12.*
		Achieve a 50% improvement in levels of adult literacy by 2015. *
Health	*Ensure that all children have access to a health clinic.*	Reduce by two-thirds the mortality rate among children under 5.
		Reduce by three-quarters the maternal mortality rate.

Actual targets are in regular type. Congruent goals are in italic type.

* Of the six goals declared at the 2000 end-of-decade conference for Education for All, this is the only one stated in quantitative terms.

in the potential role of research in achieving global goals. First, the process of inventing a "magic bullet" with a scientific imprimatur, even with a research center dedicated to a narrow research agenda, was neither straight nor short. First, the "magic bullet" was a by-product of a research center established for another purpose: the prevention, not the treatment, of cholera. The research center did not produce its raison d'être—a viable, inexpensive cholera vaccine—for several more decades. The "magic bullet" was not, therefore, immediately recognized as such; it remained to be further adapted for field use before it could be used to dramatic effect on a large scale.

Second, mixed methods of research at the invention stage of ORT played a more important role than the method that is sometimes promoted as the "gold standard" of "rigorous" scientific research: the randomized, controlled trial (RCT) (Feuer, Towne, & Shavelson, 2002). This suggests that international funders interested in encouraging scientifically based innovations might want to consider longer-term support for non-RCT research. Third, the analysis below identifies several aspects of the ORT research environment—focus, location, time, funding, international organizations, research methods, international status, and scientific status—that are not unique to microbiology, but that are not evident in any ongoing program of research in support of education in the global South.

The emphasis on Western science in this and later chapters indicates recognition rather than an uncritical endorsement of its peculiar authority in international development discourse in the last half of the 20th century and the beginning of the 21st. The Western Enlightenment values holding modern science in high esteem are part of the current culture of the world society. That culture is not immutable; at some point a great deal of agency or major eidetic or galvanizing experiences—such as the effect of the 1755 Lisbon earthquake on the Enlightenment—may shift it. But for the period under consideration here, the authority of Western science is relatively unassailable.

THE SCIENCE OF HEALTH AND EDUCATION RESEARCH

Two disciplines central to the development of individual outcome-oriented goals in public health and education serve here as exemplars of scientific research in these sectors: microbiology and cognitive neuroscience.

Although several ancient and modern disciplines underlie the current state of health sciences, research in microbiology played a particularly important role in the development of several HFA goals. Microbiology began its transformation into a systematic, modern science in the late 17th century, with the first observation of microorganisms using a crude microscope. The subdiscipline began a series of rapid advances in the second half of the 19th century as improved microscopes and related instrumentation made it possible to isolate and study ever smaller units of analysis: bacteria, cells, mitochondria, viruses. At the same time, public awareness of the germ theory of disease led to a greater appreciation of the lifesaving potential of microbiological research. Aided by ever more sophisticated instruments, complex procedures emerged to preserve and accelerate biological processes in vitro, in test tubes or petri dishes, independent of human subjects, creating a whole new arena for laboratory research.

All of this increased the legitimacy of microbiology as an exact science, in which hypotheses and counter-hypotheses could be generated, tested, and retested more quickly. Eventually, the long training necessary to learn to use sophisticated instruments in laboratories far removed from public scrutiny also contributed to the public mystification of microbiology. At the same time, periodic public successes of its work—in the form of vaccines and antibiotics administered to millions of individuals with gratifying effects—and the close ties between health research and teaching hospitals increased the authority of public health experts who attempted to bridge the divide between microbiology and public policy.

In contrast, although the history of education research sometimes traces its philosophical origins to Plato or to Jean-Jacques Rousseau's *Émile*, modern attempts to apply Western science to the study of an individual educational outcome—cognition—date only from the late 19th century, with the Progressive or New Educationists. One of the leading child psychologists and cognitive scientists of the 20th century, Jean Piaget, began his career concerned with "winning recognition, especially by his colleagues in physics and the natural sciences, for the equally *scientific* nature of the human sciences" (Munari, 1994, p. 312). Although cognitive neuroscience is arguably the most exact science to focus on education to date, precision instruments on a par with the microscope, such as functional magnetic resonance imaging (fMRIs), have only recently emerged, and their potential is still being explored.[3]

The outcome measure for cognitive neuroscience—learning—is more subtle than mortality or morbidity in microbiology. Relative to what a single blood test can reveal about the state of the body, a host of paper-and-pencil tests and performance assessments produce only crude approximations of the state of the mind of the learner. Moreover, education has multiple desired learning outcomes—learning content, learning citizenship, learning culture, learning to get along, learning to continue learning (Delors & The International Commission on Education for the Twenty-First Century, 1996; Faure & The International Commission on the Development of Education, 1972)—and consensus on objective measures of all these outcomes is not expected soon.

Without more sophisticated instruments and discrete outcome indicators; with most of its work done in public rather than in laboratories; and with a declining number of laboratory schools, cognitive scientists face more difficulty than their counterparts in microbiology in asserting their scientific jurisdiction and authority in matters pertaining to public policy. A public with lengthy personal experience in formal education systems, which tends, as a result, to assume that learning is simple and straightforward, compounds this variance, at least in industrialized countries.[4] In addition, the organization of schooling may also isolate practitioners/teachers from scientists/researchers to a greater degree in cognitive neuroscience than in microbiology.

Finally, until relatively recently, the ultimate scope of findings in microbiology was more universal than those in cognitive neuroscience. The appropriate content and target groups for education are expected to vary from place to place, as different societies define their needs in light of different social structures, physical environments, economic opportunities, history, and culture. For example, even learning such a basic foundation skill as reading varies somewhat from one context to another. Due to the idiosyncrasies of script, pronunciation, and spelling of various languages, children can become fluent readers in Italian in 1 year, whereas in English or French they may need 4 or 5 (Abadzi, 2003).

In summary, microbiological research gains much of its scientific legitimacy from its long history, exact instruments, compelling outputs, quick results, and relatively universal scope. In contrast, cognitive neuroscience, one of the more precise learning sciences, has fewer instruments to finely parse, measure, and test the various components of learning in universal terms, and its results are often highly context-specific. Efforts to make the study of learning as "scientific" as the study of microbiology are unlikely to make much progress until instrumentation in cognitive neuroscience becomes more precise. This has not, however, kept some policy researchers from trying.

"Rigor" in Scientific Research

In 2000 a group of mainly U.S. and British researchers launched the Campbell Collaboration to prepare and maintain systematic reviews of research on the effectiveness of public service interventions, including education.[5] Campbell is modeled on the Cochrane Collaboration, which since 1993 has been preparing and maintaining similar reviews of research on the effects of health interventions.[6] Researchers who wish to post reviews on the Campbell website must first submit for preapproval a draft protocol for selecting studies to be included in the review and for evaluating the evidence provided in those studies. Collaboration requirements privilege studies with experimental or randomized, controlled trial research designs[7] (Mosteller & Boruch, 2002; Torgerson & Torgerson, 2003). Experimental designs, however, tend to be expensive and used where there is some chance that development costs can later be recouped through copyrights. The education interventions that are more amenable to experimental designs include curricula and teacher training material. As of early 2014, the Campbell Collaborative database listed only nine reviews related to education, of which six were in the protocol stage.[8]

In the United States, the George W. Bush administration challenged the scientific validity of much of the nonexperimental research that had previously guided federal funding for education. At the behest of the administration, Congress passed the Education Sciences Reform Act of 2002, which created a new Institute of Education Science[9] assigned to refocus U.S. government funding on "educational practices supported by rigorous evidence," that is, experimental methods (Coalition for Evidence-Based Policy, 2003). The Center for Education at the [U.S.] National Research Council issued several warnings about unduly limiting the range of research used to inform public policy in education (National Research Council, 2002, 2004). By May 2014, the Institute's online What Works Clearinghouse had identified 77 interventions to address literacy, including 38 to improve reading comprehension for kindergarten through the end of primary grade 5 in the United States. Of these:

- 1 had positive and 18 had potentially positive effects, of which:
- 13 were supported by medium- to large-scale data, of which:
- the one positive was open-source and the other 12 were copyrighted.[10]

Beyond the United States and the United Kingdom, in 2004 the Organization for Economic Cooperation and Development held the first of four workshops to explore "evidence-based policy research in education," the first focusing on the use of RCTs.[11] A few years earlier, economists at the Abdul Jameel Latif Poverty Action Lab (f. 2003, J-PAL, Poverty Lab) associated with the Massachusetts Institute of Technology (Banerjee, Cole, Duflo, & Linden, 2003) and at the Indian Institute of Management in Ahmadabad used small-scale RCTs to evaluate low-cost education interventions in India, Kenya, and Colombia.[12]

Why do education researchers so rarely employ experimental methods (Cook, 2003)? First, as described above, in many cases, education researchers do not have the precision instruments necessary to isolate and control the phenomena of interest. Second, education interventions are typically bundled in packages that preclude studying the discrete impact of individual interventions (Weiss, 2002). Third, research since the 1960s in the United States and elsewhere has demonstrated that although teachers, classrooms, and schools can play an important role in classroom achievement, families and communities tend to play a more important one (Weiss, 2002). Therefore, the logical unit of analysis for education policy research tends to be communities, which are, by definition, too complex to be strictly comparable. For example, RCTs on certain types of peer tutoring and computer-assisted learning did increase achievement in primary mathematics in one program in India, but trials in one place alone cannot define under what conditions the same innovations would work elsewhere in other programs (Banerjee et al., 2003).

Fourth, the typical research cycle, the time elapsed between when an intervention (e.g., a new curriculum) is introduced and the desired outcome can be measured (e.g., an end-of-year exam), permits many factors to interfere with the study of the learning process (e.g., a flood that closes school for a month, transportation strikes that prevent children and teachers from attending school).

Fifth, randomized trials often come near the end of the discovery process, when small-scale and large-scale trials can be conducted on highly refined innovations with direct policy implications. Before there can be more randomized trials, there must be more basic education research and more discrete interventions.

Sixth, as previously noted, randomized field trials are expensive and few schools that develop low-cost innovations can afford to do large-scale baseline data collection and return years later to do follow-up studies. Seventh, and finally, schools and classrooms are often not willing to be randomized. For example, a child only gets one chance at 2nd grade; bad experiments during that grade can set that child's learning back for the rest of his or her school career.

Nonetheless, much education research continues in industrialized countries and, to a lesser extent, in less industrialized countries. What might be the role of nonexperimental research in identifying innovations for improving education in both types of countries until, as Weiss (2002) puts it, the random assigner comes? Research in microbiology, the foundational science for public health, is rich with suggestion, as described in the next section.

Use-Oriented Fundamental Research

The relationship between basic and applied research, or between experimental and other research methods, need not be so linear or compartmentalized. Donald Stokes urged funders of policy research to consider supporting what he called "use-oriented fundamental research" (1997) as practiced by Louis Pasteur, not, incidentally, one of history's greatest microbiologists. Stokes argued that Pasteur was equally motivated by a desire to contribute to fundamental understanding of microbiology, such as his germ theory of disease, and by a desire to find practical applications of that understanding in his own time and place, such as the means for sterilizing milk or keeping beets from turning to alcohol. This combination of interest in fundamental questions and practical applications is the hallmark of what Stokes called "use-oriented fundamental research."

In the almost 130 years since Pasteur and Koch established the germ theory of disease, many microbiologists and epidemiologists have followed their lead into "use-oriented fundamental research," employing experimental methods with careful observation and expanding fundamental science as they focused on identifying practical, situation-specific applications. Many—Schweitzer, Koch, and Walter Reed, among them—moved their research to the tropics in order to study diseases more prevalent in those climates, including malaria, cholera, and yellow fever. Although some cognitive scientists, such as Piaget, also fit into the use-oriented fundamental research category, some of the best-known education reformers in the Third World—Tagore, Freire, Illich—have adopted a more intuitive approach.

Finally, funding is always an issue. Tropical medicine was supported by the expansion of empire, explicitly in the case of Britain in Africa, less directly in the case of the United States in Panama and Southeast Asia.

During the 4 decades of the Cold War, First World governments continued strategic funding of tropical disease research at least in part to stay engaged in the affairs of the former colonies in the less industrialized world. Less Cold War funding went into education research, and education never developed a subsector equivalent to tropical medicine. In addition, health research in the less industrialized world benefited from progress in areas that were profitable to the private sector in the industrialized world. Few, if any, issues in public education in industrialized countries appear to have profit-making potential in the Third World, and private support has not been forthcoming.[13]

How do these patterns of research play out in the international development organizations that formulate global goals? I suggest the legitimacy that health researchers, in comparison with education researchers, gain from their closer proximity to Western scientific ideals enables health professionals to forge more stable communities of international experts, or "epistemic" communities (Haas, 1992). These communities are able to rationalize compromises between comprehensive and more selective approaches, and push for more outcome-oriented, coherent health policy options, such as those articulated in the Millennium Development Goals (Table 3.1, above).

A comparison of the current state of research underlying HFA and EFA might reasonably end here. However, in 2004 a research organization that played a pivotal role in the development of one magic bullet for Child Survival—oral rehydration therapy—and received the first Gates Award for Global Health (2001) for this and other efforts, at the same time it celebrated its 40th anniversary. The award and the anniversary brought together many of the early principals, prompted the compiling of oral and written histories, and brought to light some aspects of health research often missing from more conventional accounts of "scientific" advance. This material provides an unusual opportunity to observe how one research program produced a "magic bullet" for health and to consider what, if anything, this might suggest about education research and global goals.

ORAL REHDRATION THERAPY (ORT): DEVELOPING A DELIVERABLE[14]

The story below describes a fitful pattern of research over more than 110 years, during which time the discovery of a broad-spectrum treatment for diarrheal diseases was a by-product of the search for a different innovation: a cholera vaccine. International research centers in Dacca, East Pakistan (now Dhaka, Bangladesh), and Calcutta (now Kolkata), India, located in sites of frequent cholera epidemics, worked intensively beginning in the early 1960s, producing an effective treatment by 1968.

Pre-1960

The watery diarrhea[15] caused by cholera can result in severe dehydration and death in less than 24 hours. Historically endemic to Asia, cholera still erupts seasonally in Thailand, the Philippines, Bangladesh, and several other countries. When cholera epidemics in the 19th century expanded into Eastern Europe, Britain, and the United States, the search for modern preventive, curative, and palliative treatments was launched (van Heyningen & Seal, 1983).

In 1854 John Snow first associated cholera with contaminated drinking water and cut short a London epidemic with a house-to-house survey that led to a single contaminated public pump. Less than 25 years later, the cholera bacterium was identified by Pacini and reconfirmed by Koch in Calcutta, India. In the last half of the 19th century, however, the germ theory of disease brought improvements in hygiene, waste disposal, and water sanitation that reduced cholera in Europe and North America, thereby reducing demand for cholera research based on the new theory (van Heyningen & Seal, 1983).

In addition to lack of interest in the North, several scientific misunderstandings delayed by more than 100 years the development of a cholera treatment capable of success in over 95% of cases.[16] First, until the mid-20th century, most doctors assumed that the severe diarrhea and vomiting brought on by cholera injured the small intestine and that oral intake of food or liquids during diarrhea could cause further injury. Until the 1960s, therefore, starvation was part of the standard treatment for such diseases, including cholera, rendering survivors both dehydrated and malnourished and therefore more susceptible to other potentially fatal diseases (Nelson, 1985 [revised]; Ruxin, 1994).

Second, the medical community was reluctant to believe anecdotal evidence that vomiting patients could drink enough fluid (up to 20 liters per day) to mitigate cholera's dehydrating effects (Greenough, 2003). Pediatricians, not researchers, published a handful of studies in the 1950s that claimed that oral solutions containing a wide range of ingredients—carob flour, bananas, and even carrot soup—had benefited cholera patients, but these did not explain their results in terms of known physiological mechanisms (Chatterjee, 1953; Ruxin, 1994; Sack, 2003). For example, in 1953 Hemendra Nath Chatterjee published an article in the internationally respected journal *The Lancet* documenting use of an oral glucose-sodium electrolyte solution to treat 186 patients with mild to moderately severe cholera with no fatalities, a stunning result given the normally high mortality level of cholera in Bengal (Chatterjee, 1953). However, the solution was used in combination with herbal remedies peculiar to India and later researchers "generally agreed that racism or the lack of a 'scientific' rationale prevented widespread adoption of his work" (Ruxin, 1994, p. 394).

As a result, until the 1960s, the standard treatment for cholera consisted of starvation, supposedly to protect the injured gut, coupled with expensive intravenous (IV) solutions administered in hospital settings under the close supervision of health professionals trained in Western science. Such treatment was essentially unavailable to the tens of millions of cholera-affected people who lived far from modern hospitals or could not afford the only treatment offered there: intravenous saline.

The 1960s

After World War II, with ground and naval forces deployed throughout the Pacific and conflict rising in Korea and Vietnam, the U.S. government and allies funded research on cholera vaccines and treatments at several sites in Asia. In the early 1960s Capt. Robert A. Phillips, then directing the U.S. Navy Medical Research Unit II (NAMRU II), observed a previously unsuspected phenomenon: cholera patients could absorb oral saline solutions by gastric tube if glucose was added to the solutions. In 1962, Phillips's group attempted an oral therapy field trial in the Philippines based on his observation, but the solution was too concentrated, resulting in the deaths of six patients (Nelson, 1985 [revised]; Ruxin, 1994).

In 1960 the Southeast Asian Treaty Organization (1954–1977, SEATO), a coalition[17] formed by First World allies to block Second World expansion in the region, was seeking a site for a cholera research laboratory. The choice was largely between the Philippines and Pakistan and the latter, considered a weaker partner in SEATO with its western wing bordering on Communist China, was chosen in an effort to strengthen ties. In 1961 and 1962 scientists from SEATO member countries and local staff established the Pak-SEATO Cholera Research Laboratory and the Cholera Hospital in Dacca, East Pakistan (now Dhaka, Bangladesh). In 1963, scientists identified a field site with large, seasonal cholera epidemics in the Matlab subdistrict, several hours away from the city. Building on Matlab's smallpox census of 1961, the Cholera Lab set about establishing "the largest continuously operating population surveillance system in the world" (Aziz & Mosley, 1994, p. 29).

The cholera vaccine trials were expected to begin with laboratory research, and proceed to animal trials, clinical trials in the Cholera Hospital, and eventually field trials in Matlab. The deaths during the 1962 clinical trial in the Philippines translated into a very cautious approach to human trials at the Cholera Lab (Ruxin, 1994). A Technical Advisory Committee consisting of senior scientists from the United States, the United Kingdom, Australia, and the Pakistan Medical Research Council regularly reviewed the Cholera Lab's scientific agenda. Research protocols were evaluated in terms of international standards for scientific merit and ethical consideration (Henry Mosley, personal communication, June 19, 2005). Early and ongoing commitment to provide care to cholera patients when epidemics occurred, whether or not those patients were involved in field trials, engendered cooperation from the local communities in Matlab (Greenough, 2004).

Cross-cultural communication, professional competition, short-term versus lifelong commitment to the research at hand: these and other "non-scientific" issues both complicated and enriched the work at the Cholera Lab. Initially, resident expatriate scientists from the United States, Australia and the United Kingdom served for 2 or 3 years at the Cholera Lab; as time passed, through on-site training and overseas scholarships, the number of local staff and scientists grew. Many expatriates came via the U.S. National Institutes of Health (NIH, the National Institutes) and the U.S. Communicable Disease Center, now the Centers for Disease Control and Prevention (CDC, the Atlanta Center), and some continued to work on related research after they returned to the United States. Despite lack of reliable long-distance phone service, facsimile machines, and email, personal connections between staff at the Cholera Lab and these centers were close and helped to ensure better coordination than might otherwise be expected. Scientists at the Johns Hopkins International Center for Medical Research and Training in Calcutta (f. 1962, ICMRT, the Calcutta Center) at the Infectious Disease Hospital of the School of Tropical Medicine in Calcutta were working on a parallel track with the Cholera Lab, and some participants suggest that rivalry (or, in gentler terms, "exchange") stimulated scientists in both organizations to work quickly (McGrane, 2003; Nelson, 1985 [revised]). Finally, this was the Vietnam War era, and fresh faces arrived on a regular basis in the form of young American doctors who chose to enter the U.S. Public Health Service rather than be drafted into the military (Ruxin, 1994).

In order to get a gut-level understanding of cholera, newly arrived scientists were required to spend an extended internship in Matlab, and staff routinely briefed the local health community in Dacca of their progress (Greenough, 2003; Quotah, 1999; Ruxin, 1994). Thus, personal engagement with the problem was high, to the extent that one expatriate scientist, Elias Arburtyn, having contracted cholera while in the field, wrote it up as a case study in a medical journal (Cash, 2003). One of the laboratory scientists who played a major role in working out the details of the chemical composition of ORS once tried to conclude a briefing for local doctors somewhat blandly. "Oral glucose therapy," he said, "could be of value in the treatment of cholera and . . . the requirement for expensive and scarce intravenous fluids may be reduced thereby." His listeners came to different conclusions:

> One of the [tea] plantation doctors, Dr. Mackay, responded ecstatically . . . "This is one of the most profound developments in the treatment of . . . diarrhea in this century." And I remember being a little startled by that and saying to myself . . . "Gosh, maybe he's right." (Norbert Hirschhorn, quoted in Ruxin, 1994, p. 378)

Although technical supervision of the Cholera Lab from the National Institutes and CDC was close, ample funding for the Cholera Lab came, surprisingly, with few bureaucratic strings attached. In the early 1960s, at the height of the Cold War, SEATO's primary interest in funding the Cholera Lab was to keep Pakistan firmly in SEATO. One scientist recalls,

> It was literally like an open checkbook. There was no limit to the projects that could be done locally. . . . The [U.S.] State Department . . . didn't care if we did research or not. . . . If we had just done nothing but just take care of sick people that would have been enough as far as the State Department was concerned. . . . [USAID] wanted all kinds of reviewing and reporting . . . with the possibility that they might close [the Cholera Lab] if it didn't fit their agenda. [I heard second-hand] the U.S. ambassador telling [the USAID director] outright that this lab is basically to serve a political function and it is not subject to any kind of review for merit! . . . I hardly recall really working out budgets. (Mosley, 2003, p. 60)

Microbiology provided cholera researchers with a ready arsenal of instruments and measurement standards, and the cholera research itself produced more. Inexpensive "cholera cots" originally developed by Ray Watten of NAMRU II, working in Thailand during an epidemic in the 1950s, provided a simple way to measure each patient's fluid loss. The Cholera Lab and the Calcutta Center also contributed new instruments and technology, such as "Monsur's medium," named after the Bengali scientist K. A. Monsur, who designed a way to increase the speed with which cholera colonies could be identified. Working with scientists in Copenhagen, David Sachar and colleagues developed an instrument to measure the electrical charge of the small intestine, helping to establish that it did not shut down during cholera and confirming Phillips's earlier observation. In addition, as equipment in the United States rapidly improved and was replaced, the Atlanta Center and the National Institutes forwarded a steady stream of still quite up-to-date equipment to the Cholera Lab (Mosley, 2003).

Researchers learned that the chemical composition of the IV solution needed to match the composition of the fluid patients were losing. They also learned that the amount of IV solution going into a patient needed to equal the fluid lost; too much IV solution could cause congestive heart failure; too little, and the body would not rehydrate. Within a short period in the 1960s, the fatality rate for patients who arrived at the hospital severely dehydrated dropped from 30–40% to less than 1% (Ruxin, 1994).

The potential importance of oral rehydration solution as more than just a supplement to hospital-administered IV fluids dawned slowly upon a research community focused on developing a vaccine for cholera, not on treatment. The final piece in the oral rehydration therapy (ORT) puzzle fell into place in the autumn of 1967 at the Memorial Christian Hospital in Malumghat, Chittagong, on the Burma border with Bangladesh (then East Pakistan). The evening after a failed field trial, sitting in a tent, surrounded by hundreds of patients who came from villages where many more people were dying of cholera, for whom there would never be enough IV solution, one of the young public health service doctors, David Nalin, realized that one of the key protocols regarding IV solution needed to be extended to the oral solution: the patient needed to drink enough ORS to *exactly* equal the volume of fluid being lost (Nalin, 2003).

Given the failed trial in the Philippines and the generally conservative field trial environment in which the Cholera Lab operated, it was not surprising that when Nalin returned to Dacca with his insight, Phillips, now the Cholera Lab director, was initially reluctant to let staff work on clinical and field trials to test this new practical treatment. According to staff, the director was concerned that applied research would divert laboratory scientists from the "basic" research that was the principal mandate of the Cholera Lab (Ruxin, 1994). However, with support from senior scientists at partner institutions in the United States and the deputy director of the Cholera Hospital, Nalin and colleagues secured the necessary backing in late 1967 and spring 1968 for the first successful clinical trial, based on a corrected study design. Resistance to work on a treatment, rather than a vaccine, still remained, but finally, later in 1968, the young doctors were allowed to implement a large-scale, closely monitored, and ultimately successful clinical field trial with an all-oral rehydration solution.

Seasonal epidemics of cholera in Asia and in emergency settings in other regions of the world meant that the possibility of an inexpensive treatment administered by nonmedical personnel was of great interest to international organizations such as WHO and UNICEF. However, those organizations did not have a mandate to fund research and were reluctant to adopt any treatment that did not have the imprimatur of the international health community, particularly when the only difference between a liter of sugar water and an effective treatment for cholera was just a half-teaspoon of salt.

Over time, through both clinical and field trials, ORT was established as effective for a wide range of watery diarrheal diseases and, most importantly, for children as young as 1 month. Surprisingly, later research found that boiled water, while preferable, was not necessary, since most patients already had some immunity to less toxic bacteria routinely found in their drinking water. Equally importantly, researchers learned that children and adults treated early enough would instinctively drink the solution to the point of hydration, eliminating the need for medical personnel to carefully measure stool output. Finally, much later, they learned that the oral rehydration solution worked faster when administered with food.

Despite publication of the ORT studies by Cholera Lab and Calcutta Center scientists in medical journals of international repute, ORT did not immediately become the global treatment of choice for diarrheal diseases. ORT was an inexpensive, over-the-counter treatment that could be administered by family members, thereby eliminating the need for consultations with medical professionals and for the purchase of relatively expensive drugs, such as antibiotics. Pharmaceutical companies saw no profit in producing the solution, doctors were reluctant to demedicalize diarrhea, and patients couldn't believe something so simple would work. There was even some resistance within the Cholera Lab, as night nurses sometimes tried to substitute IV for oral solution to avoid the tedious work of waking up each exhausted patient every few minutes to encourage them to drink more solution (Rahman, 1994).

Like many other public health inventions, ORT might have remained unused for decades for lack of product development funds. But in 1971, East Pakistan became the site of one of the major human disasters of the last half of the 20th century and ORT was dragged out of the lab and into large-scale public service.

Out of the Laboratory and into the World

As noted earlier, the Cholera Lab was part of a larger SEATO strategy to keep Pakistan outside the sphere of influence of communist China. By early 1971, however, Pakistan was helping the United States to arrange back-channel, secret meetings between the U.S. Secretary of State and senior Chinese officials preparatory to U.S. President Richard Nixon's historic trip to China in 1972. Therefore, the United States and other SEATO members refrained from taking action in 1971, when West Pakistan rejected the outcome of an election that would have put an East Pakistan-led Socialist party in control of the Pakistan parliament. Instead, Pakistan imposed a state of emergency in the province, and sent troops with live ammunition to put down protests in Dacca.

A full-scale civil war eventually led to the deaths of more than 300,000 and the flight of more than 8 million to crowded refugee camps along the border with India. As was the case during Partition with India in 1948, minority Hindus were particular targets of attack, and they moved in disproportionate numbers into the camps. There, cholera soon broke out and mortality rates quickly reached 40%. Conscious of how little time cholera could take to spread and kill millions, and with no alternative mass treatment in hand, medical teams from the Calcutta Center mixed large batches of the dry ingredients of rehydration solution and sent them to the camps with instructions to mix them with drinking water or, lacking that, river water with the sediment removed. The solution was distributed with brief instructions to refugees who, with little medical supervision, administered it to their relatives. The mortality rate from cholera in the camps supervised by the Calcutta Center subsequently fell to less than 5% (Mahalanabis, Choudhury, Bagchi, Bhattacharya, & Simpson, 1973).

Scientific evidence of efficacy under the most difficult conditions, published in the most highly respected, peer-reviewed international medical journal, still did not lead to rapid, widespread acceptance and use of ORT. ORT was indeed a "magic bullet" deliverable—low-cost, low-tech, scientifically endorsed, with a compelling, widely accepted outcome measure—but it was in need of a gun. The components of this "gun" included a communication campaign, a delivery system, access to the highest levels of power where national political commitment could be secured, and, given oral rehydration therapy's nonexistent profit margin, public funds.

Ten years later, ORT was not among the cases highlighted by the reports prepared in preparation for the 1978 Alma-Ata conference. Just a year later, ORT featured prominently at a Bellagio meeting as a low-cost treatment for the infectious disease responsible for more deaths in the Third World than any other (Walsh & Warren, 1979). Within 2 years, Jon Rohde, a young American doctor who had fulfilled his public service working on ORT in Bangladesh, would find an open door at UNICEF, where Grant would, at least for a while, champion ORT as the best hope for child survival.

ORT is now recommended by international health organizations, the American Academy of Pediatricians, and the Atlanta Centers, and represents a significant transfer of technology from the Third to the First and Second Worlds. Ironically, oral rehydration salts are now widely available in inexpensive packets in almost every country except the United States, the Cholera Lab's largest funder (Santosham, Keenan, Jim, Broun, & Glass, 1997). Without a patent and with such simple ingredients, no drug company in the United States considers it profitable to produce ORS packets, particularly now, when the formula for a homemade version is available free on the Internet.[18]

HEALTH RESEARCH: LESS HEAT, MORE LIGHT

In the hot war of words and funding around education research and evaluation methods, the invention of oral rehydration provides some ammunition for mixed-methods partisans. In many ways, research at the Cholera Lab and the Calcutta Center was both basic and applied and therefore has many of the hallmarks of Stokes's "use-oriented fundamental research" (1997). As the ORT case demonstrates, the invention of such an intervention involved many types of research, tightly focused on a single disease, in close proximity to where that disease was most prevalent, with lavish support not tied to a 5-year funding cycle, and with the blessing and support of respected international public health research centers.

Proximity

A Cholera Lab alumnus who later taught at the Harvard School of Public Health declared, "Most of research is asking questions, and you ask better questions in the field" (Richard Cash, personal communication, June 25, 2005). Many accounts by laboratory alumni (International Centre for Diarrheal Disease Research, Bangladesh, 2003) refer to an article by a laboratory scientist, "Taking Science Where the Diarrhea Is" (Rohde & Northrup, 1976). The site where the final piece of the oral rehydration puzzle—that the amount of solution consumed should equal the bodily fluids being lost through diarrhea and vomiting—occurred to a laboratory scientist was a missionary hospital in the midst of a cholera epidemic. Nonetheless, few scientists foresaw the potential mass applications of oral rehydration, and those applications did not emerge until the Calcutta Center was confronted with the massive 1971 epidemic in refugee camps along the border of India and East Pakistan.

Time

The transformation of rehydration therapy from an expensive treatment delivered in a sterile setting, where medical professionals carefully calibrated fluid input and output every 4 hours, into a solution that could be dispensed by family members in refugee camps using whatever water was at hand was not accomplished in a year or two by visiting consultants. It drew on more than 100 years of instrumentation and involved 6 years of full-time work for dozens of researchers in several research centers; more than a decade of surveys and field trials to move the preparation of rehydration solution from laboratories to rural homes (Chowdhury & Cash, 1996); and a further decade to be reproduced in other high-priority countries.[19] No such discrete component of EFA benefits from such a sustained program of use-oriented fundamental research, product development, and/or marketing research in any international institution in any less industrialized country today.

Funding

Interest in funding research on cholera ebbed at the end of the 19th and the beginning of the 20th century as the disease became less of a threat to the industrialized world. Later in the 20th century, the Cold War gave cholera research a boost. SEATO members, including Australia, the United Kingdom, and the United States, were interested in a cholera vaccine to keep their troops healthy in the event of military action in the region. SEATO wanted to use members' technical assistance, proceeds from the sale of U.S. food aid, and surplus equipment from members' scientific laboratories to help tie Pakistan to the First World; East Pakistan just happened to be a good research site for cholera. This windfall of resources with few strings attached was relatively serendipitous and was not the result of more rational planning and allocation of research funds by international organizations working in the health sector, such as the chronically underfunded WHO. Later funding for the successors to the Cholera Lab would benefit from long-term investments from the Rockefeller and other foundations.

Similarly, as the specter of mass illiteracy ebbed in the postindustrial world at the end of the 20th century, interest in and funding for research on this and other education issues more relevant to the less industrialized world stagnated. In the 1990s, population growth concerns, tangentially related to First World security, translated into more funding for girls' education. After 2001, the War on Terror began providing more development assistance for education projects in less industrialized Muslim countries than ever before, including more for girls' education. The War on Terror has not, however, provided more funds for a long-term education research program undertaken by an international center located in the Third World.

Research Methods

For ORT, randomized field trials came at strategic points in 100-plus years of research. Throughout that period researchers developed many measurement tools and repeatedly tested promising interventions, or some component of them, in limited settings. Early effective treatments for cholera, such as carrot soup, were not systematically developed and measured. Their inventors could not explain in Western scientific terms the mechanisms by which they worked, and the treatments did not diffuse. At the Cholera Lab, once ORT was invented, RCTs in the late 1960s and 1970s were the primary research method used to prove the efficacy of various formulations and to determine dosage. However, both up to and following ORT's invention, qualitative and nonexperimental studies played the leading role in identifying possible directions for research and how treatments might be adapted to increase acceptance and use (David Sack, personal communication June 23, 2005).

International Status and Support

The Cholera Lab was created with close ties to respected international health research and teaching centers in the United States and later established working relationships with similar centers in other countries. These ties brought expertise, equipment, informal second opinions, rigorous institutional review, training and exchange opportunities for long-term Bengali staff, publication opportunities, and a broader audience for the Cholera Lab's findings. A steady stream of researchers involved in a wide range of tropical diseases continues to use Matlab as a field site, now with more than 40 years of data for tens of thousands of subjects.

Several institutes for educational research have been operating in less industrialized countries for decades. While many of these have the sort of close backward linkages (to the grass roots) that Bell (1987) suggested at the end of Chapter 2, these institutes lack forward linkages to highly reputed international research centers. They also lack the sort of multinational scientific support and long-term foundation funding enjoyed by the Cholera Lab, now the Center for Health and Population Research.

Scientific Status

Articles on ORT began appearing in respected international journals, such as *The Lancet*, within a year of its first successful clinical trial. Over time, the development of a diarrheal disease specialization within public health also lent more scientific status to later ORT research. Researchers based in laboratories in the First World, however, won the Nobel Prize for discovering the underlying biological process that made ORS work. Those conducting the fundamental use-oriented research that led to the discovery of ORS did not.

Death Focuses the Mind

Cholera can lead to death in less than 24 hours and ORT can reverse the course of the disease in just a few hours. Few interventions are as immediately compelling as ORT, yet even so, this innovation was not immediately adopted worldwide.

CONCLUSIONS

This chapter explored the origins of one key innovation that advanced Child Survival. The analysis does not resolve the fundamental incommensurability of the desired outcomes in the two sectors—the relative simplicity of eradicating a specific toxin from the human body versus the complexity of providing a child with 5 or 6 years of basic education—but it highlights roads not taken by education researchers that are worth revisiting.

The first half of this chapter compared microbiology and cognitive science as exemplars of scientific specialties relevant to the advance of global health and education goals, respectively. In the process, many of the well-known reasons why scientific research in the health sector has produced more universal innovations in support of global goals than in the education sector came to the fore. Microbiology has an advance of a century or two on cognitive science in terms of measurement and in terms of interest from the most generous source of governmental funding, security.

The second half of the chapter showed that RCTs played a minor role in the invention of one magic bullet for Child Survival in the 1960s. Indeed, much of the normal science that did advance this magic bullet is within the realm of education research. Measurement was particularly important in the early stages of cholera research. Tracking the progress of the disease and its response to various interventions at a cellular level was the foundation of the laboratory and clinical research. Innovations in measurement were necessary before comparisons between control and treatment groups could be designed. Clearly, education could benefit from better systematic measurement. Equally clearly, an international research center, staffed with international researchers and closely tied to strong education research centers worldwide, would also probably speed along the development of appropriate measurement. On the other hand, the bias of world culture toward universal and quantitative measurement, suggested in several propositions in Chapter 1, is driving Third World countries to join large-scale cross-national assessments developed in the global North. Unintentionally, however, these expensive assessments may divert limited national psychometric and statistical expertise from the diverse types of research needed to develop interventions to improve the quality of education and to closely study their implementation. Therefore, broader participation in large-scale, cross-national assessments is no substitute for close, long-term associations with respected international research centers that can provide technical assistance to set priorities with a much broader research agenda and to help execute them.

Similarly, demanding measurement for accountability too soon can stifle innovation. Through its association with security-oriented SEATO, scientists working at the Cholera Lab in the 1960s did not have to justify their many small projects in advance in terms of results-based frameworks that defined what they would discover and when. SEATO did not demand full-scale evaluations in 5 years or less. However, after 1971, a larger share of the budget of the Cholera Lab and the research center that succeeded it came from diverse international donors, all of which expected a larger role in the direction and monitoring of that center. These international donors demanded that the research center adopt blueprints and scripts relating to scientific research protocols and international development discourse, including sustainability, local participation, and the rights of patients and research subjects. All of these subjects were of concern to Cholera Lab scientists in the 1960s, but these required far fewer formal reviews from far fewer funders and technical oversight boards. Looking back, all of these scientists suggest that current protocols would have significantly slowed their work in the 1960s.

The invention of ORT lends support to at least two earlier *propositions about the role of organizations* in the process of launching and sustaining global initiatives, and also suggests several others.

> O2.14. Global initiatives with angel investors will proceed more
> quickly than those without.

The role of the military-oriented SEATO as an "angel" investor in the case of the Cholera Lab was no more ironic than the role played by the Rockefeller Foundation, created by capitalist "robber barons," in the founding of a half-dozen international agriculture research centers beginning in the 1960s. Although Rockefeller was a supporter of the internationalization of the Cholera Lab and Rockefeller's International Education Board took an early interest in mass education in Africa, neither that foundation nor any other has come forward to fund an international center for research for education in the global South.

> O2.15. Global initiatives will proceed more quickly when a
> charismatic innovator or early adopter is well positioned in an
> organization that has a formal or informal mandate to act in the
> domain of the initiative.

Cholera Lab histories (Nelson, 1985; Ruxin, 1994) identify several champions well placed in the research centers that provided oversight for the lab, such as the U.S. National Institutes of Health and the U.S. Centers for Disease Control. In addition, several Cholera Lab alumni also took it upon themselves to build and follow up on ORT trials (see Chapter 6), carrying ORT to other contexts and countries.

Participants in the early ORT research insist that locating the Cholera Lab in a country and a field site with regular, devastating outbreaks of cholera speeded the work, suggesting a new generalization relating to the functioning of research centers as organizations.

> O3.1. Research centers working in close proximity to the problem in need of their attention will develop better research questions and innovations faster than those working at some remove from the areas of greatest need.

Location alone, however, is not enough. For example, an international education research center now based in the Philippines has some parallels to the Cholera Lab. The Southeast Asian Ministers of Education Organization (f. 1965, SEAMEO), like SEATO, began as a First World effort to shore up relations in the region during the Vietnam War. Unlike SEATO, however, SEAMEO early on diversified its funders and members and became a regionally directed effort (Cummings, 1986b). SEAMEO has established more than a dozen regional centers for research and training, including one for educational innovations and technology (f. 1970, INNOTECH). INNO-TECH could not develop close ties and exchanges with many world-class centers of excellence in education research because, sadly, they were hard to find. INNOTECH's funding was modest compared to the Cholera Lab's, and the innovation hailed as its most promising, Instructional Management by Parents, Communities, and Teachers (1974, IMPACT), never scaled up significantly in any of the six countries where it was eventually attempted, including Bangladesh (Nielsen & Cummings, 1999).

Finally, the case demonstrates that those conducting use-oriented fundamental research, like the Cholera Lab scientists, will not necessarily be the first to understand its potential, like the local doctors from the tea plantations. Scientific research institutes are good places for inventing and testing innovations for basic efficacy, but they may not be the best place to adapt them for use and to deliver them to areas of greatest demand. How do delivery systems get developed, and by whom?

Adapting

A Tale of Two Sectors

Colette Chabbott and Mushtaque Chowdhury

The First Law of the Conservation of Social Energy:
Of the people principally involved [in successful projects] . . . most . . . had previously participated in other, generally more "radical" *experiences of collective action that had generally not achieved their objective,* often because of official repression.

—Albert Hirschman (1984, pp. 42–43, emphasis added)

The preceding chapter proposed that embedding scientific research in an environment surrounded by pressing human need can, in some cases, accelerate the discovery of scientific innovations to address that need. The Pak-SEATO Cholera Research Laboratory (PS-CRL, the Cholera Lab), engaging in use-oriented fundamental research and also responding to frequent cholera outbreaks, expanded its mandate beyond the search for a vaccine for soldiers and invented a new, cheaper, quicker, and better treatment. The Cholera Lab's sterile approach to oral rehydration, however, although able to serve more patients than an intravenous approach, still wasn't practical for the vast majority of cholera sufferers in rural East Pakistan, much less in other countries. Nor was the Cholera Lab able to move quickly to adapt ORT to village conditions or to translate research results into something easy to understand for those most in need. This kind of action research (Lewin, 1958) and social mobilization called for a very different kind of organization: field-based, quick-responding, ready to learn by trial and error.

This chapter describes how one such organization with these capacities emerged in the 1970s following the War of Independence in Bangladesh. After years of looking for ways to help provide health services in rural areas, the Bangladesh NGO BRAC took just a few months to adapt the Cholera Lab's oral rehydration solution into something that illiterate families could make from ingredients readily available in the most remote villages, under the most unsterile conditions. More to our point, the same organization, about a decade later, based on its success with oral rehydration, set about transforming an adult functional education model into a 3-year basic education course for children that, for a while, became the talk of EFA. This chapter highlights many parallels between the two interventions at the adaptation stage, which in our terms covers both field experiments and small-scale pilots.

BANGLADESH AND BRAC

As explained in Chapter 1, soon after its independence in 1971 Bangladesh was labeled a "basket case." However offensive the metaphor, few at the time disputed the gravity of the situation that prompted it. In its first 2 years as an independent country, Bangladesh suffered a cyclone, a famine, and two smallpox epidemics.[1] At independence, at least 70% of Bangladeshis—more than 35 million people—were living below the poverty line without a social safety net. More than 80% of them were in rural areas, but of these, the vast majority were landless and depended upon wage labor and micro-enterprises to survive. Rural literacy rates were less than 20%. Rural primary schools charged fees in excess of what most rural families could pay and accommodated less than half of rural children. Health services were also unevenly distributed; the ratio of doctors to inhabitants in urban areas was 1:1,500, in rural areas, 1:40,000. Outside cities, most general hospital beds were in a handful of private hospitals, the majority operated by Christian missionaries (Loomis, 1976).

Despite the limited scope of education and health services and their largely private provision up to that time, the 1972 Bangladesh Constitution assigned to the state responsibility for supplying a uniform and universal system of education and improving the general state of public health. In 1973 the government of Bangladesh launched a series of 5-year plans to address these and other constitutional mandates. Three years after the launching, however, a U.S. Public Health Service-funded study concluded:

> Given Bangladesh's extremely limited resource base, the attempt to create a comprehensive rural health system with supporting facilities and trained personnel in five years, is simply not feasible. In 1975, almost halfway through the plan's period, very little had been done regarding the implementation of the broad health objectives outlined in 1973. This governmental inaction can be attributed to four factors:

- The lack of an operational plan, which clearly delineates a specific goal-oriented program.
- Lack of efficient administrative mechanism.
- Lack of national resources—financial as well as manpower.
- Lack of governmental commitment to the health sector.

Any of these four factors could seriously damage implementation of a health policy; combined, they make it totally impossible to implement. (Loomis, 1976, p. 44)

Indeed, the government provided little basic health, much less education, services in many rural areas during the first 2 decades of independence. Donors, particularly those preoccupied with the looming population crisis, such as USAID, were anxious to fund health and family planning activities through whatever organizations proved themselves the most effective. NGOs, both international and local, began experimenting with health service delivery.

The Bangladesh Rehabilitation Assistance Committee, later simply known as BRAC, was one of the up-and-coming national NGOs. BRAC was founded by several Bengali friends, including Fazle Hasan Abed, to help provide relief for refugees in camps along the border with India during the 1971 war and later to help those refugees resettle in the particularly hard-hit Hindu areas of Sulla, Sylhet district.

It was the second foray into nongovernmental action for this group. After the 1970 cyclone, the Pakistan government neglected to respond to a natural disaster that left more than a half a million dead and millions homeless in East Pakistan. Abed, then the chief accountant for Shell Oil Company in the southern port city of Chittagong, East Pakistan, offered his house as an organizing point for those anxious to provide relief for survivors. Many Bengali and expatriate friends, such as doctors and wives associated with the Cholera Lab and priests from Notre Dame College in Dhaka, led the effort (Rohde, 2014). In the midst of this extreme emergency, they drew up detailed plans for rehabilitation for an island with 13,000 survivors; in response to a proposal for about US$380,000, Bread for the World promised about US$800,000.

During the 1971 war, Abed resigned from his position with Shell and lobbied in London to win more support for the liberation effort and, working with Bengali friends, to raise money for refugee relief. After the war, Abed returned to Dacca and worked with his friend Viquar Choudhury to convert some of the proceeds from the sale of his house in London into relief programs for Sulla. In March 1972, a French journalist wrote of this area:

The village of Derai is a commercial center. . . . All along our route there was the spectacle of villages burned to the ground. Only the hard earth foundations remained where the returned refugees . . . were trying to build straw shelters that would not even protect them from the sun, let alone the rain. . . . A hailstorm of rare violence for the season . . . drenched the inside of their houses, food was laid out to dry on oozing mats, [there was] indescribable desolation and women in tears, pleading with BRAC staff to give them materials to rebuild their houses right away. (Chen, 1983, p. 1)

Young, nationalistic youth inspired by the success of the War of Liberation formed the backbone of a temporary relief organization.[2] BRAC delivered clothing and food, purchased and floated massive rafts of bamboo poles for use in house-building, and brought twine for fishing nets and many other materials the returnees needed to restart their lives. With its first grant from Oxfam, BRAC established a pattern of overperforming, building more than 14,000 houses instead of the planned 10,500.

In October 1972, BRAC submitted an ambitious 2-year plan to Oxfam for integrated rural development in an area of about 160 square miles. This plan included organizing 200-plus primary cooperative societies for farmers and fishermen, reaching the entire adult population of the area (about 84,000) with literacy classes, and enrolling all children in primary school. In hindsight, this was clearly a case of a new energetic organization biting off more than it could chew, scaling up too fast. Many young organizations might have collapsed under the weight of this "failure." However, BRAC submitted a candid report to its donors. As had been the case during the 1970 cyclone, those donors lacked alternative organizations with a track record for reaching the most needy, and they continued supporting BRAC (Smillie, 2009).

In 1971, there were no road maps for how to work in such remote areas with so few resources. Just 4 years after its founding, BRAC created a Research and Evaluation Division (f. 1975, RED, BRAC Researchers) to supplement the field staff's action research efforts and to carry out more and larger surveys. Two years later, one of the group's first and most compelling findings was that, in the communities where BRAC was working, the benefits of its efforts were accruing disproportionately to better-off and elite community members.[3] This was the first of many instances where BRAC researchers would reveal a fundamental flaw with an approach into which the organization had invested significant, sometimes years, of effort. Far from abandoning the approach, in many cases BRAC made radical reforms, out of which emerged some significant successes. As a result, beginning in 1977, BRAC stopped organizing its work around communities and began organizing the relatively more disadvantaged and marginalized into cooperative groups. Inspired by Paulo Freire (1970), BRAC aimed to raise consciousness in these groups about who got what and why, and to initiate group activities that might change resource distribution patterns, beginning with basic literacy and numeracy skills.

BRAC: LEARNING BEFORE *LOBON-GUR*

Less than 10 years after its founding, BRAC was featured in a major compilation of promising approaches to rural community-based development (Ahmed, 1980). By that time, BRAC itself had developed a "learning approach" that would attract much attention in the international development literature in the years to come (Ahmed, Chabbott, Joshi, & Pande, 1993; Chen, 1983; Korten, 1980; Lovell, 1992; Rohde, 2005a; Zaman & Karim, 2005). Among other sources, BRAC's learning approach drew on the notion of "action research." Kurt Z. Lewin described the process this way: "Rational social management proceeds in a spiral of steps, each of which is composed of a circle of planning, action, and fact-finding about the result of action" (1958, p. 201).

Needs in rural Bangladesh were legion in the 1970s and remain daunting today. Determining what interventions would make the most difference for the largest number of people and, of those, which were within BRAC's capacities to support has been and continues to be one of the organization's core tasks. That task was closely tied to an assessment of what sort of staff could be found in or persuaded to live near the remote places that needed the most help, which interventions those particular staff had the capacity to deliver, and how much support BRAC could muster for them.

Matching Up Deliverables and Delivery Agents

During its first year of working with the refugees, BRAC had determined that 10 to 15 diseases accounted for 95% of the cases that came to the attention of their health staff.[4] In 1972, while the new government was preparing its first 5-year plan and health strategy, BRAC fielded four physicians to provide outpatient services in four clinics free of charge to all residents of Sulla. Within a year it was evident that these doctors reached far too few patients. About that time, the rest of the world was becoming interested in the rural "barefoot doctors" working in China.[5] BRAC's next move, therefore, was to train locally recruited men to serve as paramedics who would treat minor illnesses for a small fee and refer more complex cases to doctors at the clinics. Nine months of theoretical and practical training for the paramedics covered nutrition, child care, basic public health, family planning, and 2 weeks at the Cholera Research Lab. The training also included an orientation to "essential drugs" necessary to treat the 13 conditions BRAC health staff had identified as most prevalent and amenable to simple treatment.

From a list of 72 applicants, BRAC chose 21 trainees, of whom only 11 completed the course. High levels of dropouts or dismissals were common during BRAC's early years, as many early recruits did not understand the volume of work and diligence that BRAC would demand of them. One senior BRAC manager joined the organization as a new Dhaka University graduate where he had been a member of the Communist Party. Of his first assignment with BRAC, he said:

> It was the first time in my life I had seen really poor people. As students [and members of the Communist Party], we went to the villages and spoke to poor people, but they were not the really poor people. As someone from the urban higher middle class, when I saw people living in a house with a tin roof, I thought they were poor. But they were not. They were actually better off. In Rowmari I changed my view . . . of all that [Communist] talk. They were not working with the poor people at all; now I was seeing poor people for the first time. (M. Aminul Alam, quoted in Smillie, 2009, p. 60)

The training was revised in light of the 1st year of experience, and 20 out of 42 trainees completed a 6-month paramedic course in August 1974, at which point BRAC concluded it could cover Sulla with one paramedic for every five to seven villages or about 5,000 people (Rohde, 2005c).

Trying to foster self-reliance, BRAC experimented with various approaches to cost recovery in its health programs. For example, paramedics sold essential medicines at cost, except in cases where prolonged treatment was beyond the patient's means. They also charged a minimum consultation fee, but even this was too much for half of the population. BRAC experimented with group health insurance schemes, but there BRAC ran into a factor that would shape most of its work in rural Bangladesh: those most in need were not willing or able to pay for anything in advance. As in BRAC's other community-oriented activities, the poorest were not well served by the health program. Moreover, some paramedics had begun posing as doctors, dispensing drugs and offering treatments beyond their training in order to earn more money. After 4 years the insurance scheme was abandoned and support to the paramedics ceased.

Women as Delivery Agents

BRAC's struggles with male health workers forced it to look more closely at what women might be able to do in rural communities. Both maternal and infant mortality rates were high in rural areas, and BRAC early on recognized that attending births and discussing birth control and breast-feeding, at least in a culture that tried to segregate by gender, were not jobs that men could do. However, at least initially, most traditional birth attendants, or *dais*, were not interested in whatever training BRAC was offering. A history of the early years of BRAC's health program reported, "*Dais* were bound to tradition, hard to train, and did not follow directions as given" (Zaman & Karim, 2005, p. 39).

BRAC struggled for years to find effective ways to employ rural women as health care delivery agents. Of the 100 lessons in BRAC's functional literacy curriculum for adult groups, seven soon focused on problems associated with large families and possible solutions through family planning. In January 1974, BRAC established four fully equipped clinics with qualified male and female staff providing all family planning services, including vasectomies, free of charge. In addition, BRAC was learning that word-of-mouth and face-to-face interactions were the most effective means of communication in illiterate communities. However, families preferred that women remain in their family compounds and did not permit outside men to enter. BRAC therefore experimented with a new cadre of Lady Family Planning Organizers, each responsible for registering all couples of child-bearing age in her village, going house to house motivating those couples to enroll in family planning clinics, delivering contraceptive supplies to those who enrolled, and referring clients to family planning clinics as complications arose. Acceptance of modern contraceptives was soon much higher in the poor, rural areas where BRAC was working (20%) than in the country as a whole (7%), and BRAC achieved a higher continuation rate of contraceptive users than any other similar project at the time in Bangladesh.[6]

Finding other roles for women besides family planning and maternal health took longer. The best statistics at the time suggested that Bangladesh's infant mortality rate was 150:1,000 live births, and children up to 4 years old accounted for 40% of all deaths (Loomis, 1976). BRAC's surveys showed that the situation in Sulla was much worse. About 60% of all ailments that had been treated by male paramedics were for common diseases, such as diarrhea, dysentery, scabies, fever, and intestinal worms. These data contributed to BRAC's decision to phase out male paramedics and phase in *Shasthya Shebikas (Shebikas)*, the village women who would become the main delivery agent for BRAC's health program. Each of BRAC's disadvantaged groups chose a *Shebika* from among their female members, who was then trained to provide many of the services previously provided by Family Planning Organizers and paramedics. By selling medicines purchased at cost from BRAC to community members for a 10% markup and charging a small consulting fee (less for group members, more for others in the village), the *Shebika* became self-sustaining. At the same time, her membership in the group made her more accountable and less likely to expand her business into areas where she was not qualified.

The *Shebika* model did not scale-up immediately because success was mixed and BRAC had learned from the Family Planning Organizer program that "individuals will not necessarily limit their family size until certain basic needs are met: health services, employment, social and economic security" (Chowdhury & Chowdhury, 1978, p. 273). The *Shebika* approach was finally implemented on a large scale when BRAC had an integrated Rural Development Program in thousands of villages, about a decade later.

A timeline of the history of BRAC's early health programs illustrates its trial-and-error approach: of a dozen or so milestones in its first 7 years, BRAC includes five that represent partial or complete failures. These failures include: traditional birth attendants refused to be trained; TB program suffered high dropout rates; a flood forced cancellation of premiums for a health insurance program; some of the village paramedics reverted to being quacks; and the male *Shebikas* did not work out (Rohde, 2005b).

From these early years, BRAC's health program learned several major lessons (Zaman & Karim, 2005). First, their target group was preeminently concerned with their socioeconomic condition, not health. Given a choice, the poor invested first in income-generating activities; only after they perceived an improvement in their socioeconomic condition would they consider spending on preventive health care or health insurance. In many cases, target groups would need to be motivated to adopt some health innovation, the more so if there was a cost associated with the innovation and its benefits were not immediate and overwhelming. Change at the community level often needed a change agent to provide motivation and support. Second, Family Planning Organizers and *Shebikas* could provide fewer services than a fully trained paramedic, but they had a better chance of improving health by virtue of providing more essential services to more women. It was possible to get better results from a fully implemented modest set of interventions than a more complete, complex set.

Third, soon after independence, the government adopted a health services strategy that focused on preventive care.[7] As government rural health clinics slowly began appearing in rural areas, BRAC health workers spent less time on direct delivery of health service and more on helping the most disadvantaged gain access to government health services. To these lessons, Martha Chen (1983), with Ayesha Abed, Abed's wife, the first codirector of BRAC's women's program, would add the centrality of women, both as village-level workers and as the principal target group for BRAC's organizing efforts. All of these lessons carried over into BRAC's oral rehydration and primary education programs and speeded their rollout, as described below.

ADAPTING ORAL REHYDRATION SOLUTION (ORS):
TESTING THE *LOBON-GUR* SOLUTION[8]

Several years after the refugees' return to Sulla, cholera and other diarrheal diseases were still the major cause of death. Frequent bouts of diarrhea from cholera and other common diseases, such as *rotavirus* and *E. coli*, stunted many children and left them more vulnerable to other potentially fatal endemic diseases such as measles.

Ongoing research at the Cholera Lab and elsewhere had determined that ORS was effective for all forms of diarrhea, even in very young children, and was more effective when combined with food. By the late 1970s, international health researchers had developed and tested dry packets of salt and sugar that could be mixed with drinking water for use at home without medical supervision. However, given the poor state of communications and transportation and the low levels of literacy in rural Bangladesh, the likelihood that such packets would reach and be effectively used in the rural areas that needed it most, such as Sulla, was low. In 1978 the Cholera Lab had become the International Center for Diarrheal Disease Research, Bangladesh (ICDDR,B, the Diarrhea Center), and remained actively involved in many types of ORT research. "The scientific director [of the Diarrhea Center], Dr. Lincoln Chen, felt strongly that, even if sufficient quantities of ORS [packets] could be produced, packaged and marketed, poor people, especially in remote areas, would not have access to it" (Lovell & Abed, 1993, p. 217).

The *Lobon-Gur* Solution: The Field Experiment

By 1978, BRAC had learned a lot about health problems at the village level, had devised potential interventions to address several of them, and was experimenting with delivery agents. However, an intervention that could quickly improve the health of its members and that was within its organizational capacities to deliver remained elusive. In 1979, at a monthly project meeting in Sulla, Abed and field managers discussed what BRAC might do to contribute to the International Year of the Child, particularly what activity might have the biggest impact on the infant mortality rate. Immunization, for example, was not a possibility; many jurisdictions in Bangladesh still lacked electricity, and the cold chain—a way of keeping vaccines cold in the field—wasn't yet available. They concluded that teaching women how to make and administer a simple oral rehydration solution in their own homes would be the most cost-effective and rapid way to reduce infant mortality (Chowdhury & Cash, 1996).

At that time WHO did not encourage home-available nonstandardized rehydration solution, especially if it was formulated with just sugar and salt, without other electrolytes such as potassium and bicarbonate (Cutting, 1977, quoted in Chowdhury & Cash, 1995). In the United States, efforts to train groups of nurses failed to produce a consistently safe solution from a few basic ingredients. From this, many concluded that only highly trained professionals could be entrusted with the task.

The leadership at BRAC, however, drew very different conclusions from the U.S. research. From its own work BRAC had become convinced that one-time preservice training, such as that given to the U.S. nurses, was rarely effective. Almost all of BRAC's staff received on-the-job mentoring and monitoring in addition to preservice training. Moreover, 7 years after independence, there weren't enough quacks, let alone medical professionals, in Sulla or other rural areas to address large-scale, annual outbreaks of cholera and other endemic, potentially fatal diarrheal diseases. BRAC concluded that experience in the refugee camps strongly suggested that family members could dispense ORS and that too many lives were at stake not to attempt a stopgap, though imperfect, solution.

The *Lobon-Gur* Solution: Adapting ORS to the Rural Context

If training women to make ORS appeared a smaller problem in rural Bangladesh than it might elsewhere, measurement was a bigger issue. Poor, rural households had few cooking or eating utensils. The proportions of salt, sugar, and water in ORS had to be exact not just to be effective, but also to avoid potentially fatal concentrations of salt. The water measurement problem was resolved when researchers discovered that approximately 90% of women in Sulla could estimate a *seer*, a measurement used in daily cooking equal to approximately a liter, to within 25% of a half-liter (Ellerbrock, 1981). Measuring the appropriate amount of dry ingredients was more challenging. By trial and error, working in his own kitchen, Abed combined two ingredients available in almost all rural households—salt (*lobon*) and unrefined sugar (*gur*)—using fistfuls and two- and three-finger pinches, resulting in a prototype for a consistent, effective *lobon-gur* solution.

Since the principal advantage of the *lobon-gur* solution lay in the availability of all necessary ingredients in almost all rural households, the deliverable in this field experiment would not be the *lobon-gur* solution. Instead, BRAC's deliverable was an educational message covering how to make the *lobon-gur* solution, when to use it, how to manage children's nutrition afterward, and how to prevent diarrhea in the future. Since mothers, daughters, and mothers-in-law provided most of the child care in Bangladesh, these women were identified as the target group.

Identifying Delivery Agents and Maintaining Quality Control

The delivery system for the message required the most innovation. In the 1970s, radio was not widely available in Bangladesh, and gathering mothers in a central training location was not practical in rural areas where women were discouraged from appearing in public. Women would have to be trained individually, in their homes, and, given high illiteracy rates, face-to-face. Moreover, this training would have to be delivered by women of good repute who could enter houses and move between villages. Finally, because the margin of error between an effective solution and one dangerously high in salt was narrow, a system for monitoring how well the target group could make and use the solution had to be devised. In this way, the program identified and retrained households—or Rehydration Workers—that were making or using *lobon-gur* inappropriately.

Most of the learning came from implementation in the field. BRAC conducted its first field experiment in two villages sufficiently close to BRAC's local office so that the program supervisor and two female oral rehydration workers could meet every day to share experiences and work to improve the protocol. An American volunteer doctor drafted the first trial messages, and the workers were trained to deliver the messages face-to-face to individual mothers. The same expatriate doctor, assisted by a local paramedic, maintained quality control, visiting a village several days after the oral rehydration team had left, asking mothers to make some *lobon-gur* solution, and sending some of these solutions by special courier to the Diarrhea Center for analysis.

From the earliest days, results were reported not just to donors but to the international scientific community. By 1980, the results from a representative sample of women trained under this field experiment were collected and published in the international journal *Tropical Doctor*: 87% of the randomly chosen women could make an effective solution; 11.5% made an ineffective solution; 1.1% made a solution that was potentially dangerous; and 0.4% made a dangerous solution (Ellerbrock, 1981). Considering the high mortality rate for untreated cholera in rural areas, the results, though not based on a randomized controlled trial, were compelling.

For BRAC, the 3-month field experiment demonstrated proof of concept. It showed that:

- Illiterate women could learn to make an effective *lobon-gur* solution.
- Young women with 8 to 10 years of education could be effective trainers for making and administering *lobon-gur* solution.
- A cost-effective monitoring system could determine how much mothers absorbed of the *lobon-gur* solution lesson and how the training might be improved.

- Necessary management and logistics—such as shipping sample solutions to the Diarrhea Center—were feasible (Chowdhury & Cash, 1996).

In addition to hundreds of trained mothers, the field experiment produced a refined message—"10 Points to Remember" (Table 4.1)—that, properly delivered by a trained Rehydration Worker, could communicate the definition of diarrhea, the way to make and use *lobon-gur* solution to treat it, and some nutritional advice, all in about 20 minutes.

Oral Therapy Program (OTP): Piloting on a Large Scale

Encouraged by the results of the field experiment and already beginning to expand other rural development programs beyond Sulla, BRAC began discussing a larger pilot project, the Oral Therapy Program (1979–80, OTP). A larger-scale pilot in Sulla and in two neighboring subdistricts would help BRAC decide whether the *lobon-gur* solution training could be expanded into areas where BRAC had no other programs. Such a pilot could also help resolve delivery support issues such as: how to organize training for large numbers of new staff; how to arrange food and lodging for the staff in the field; and how to pay them without having to travel with or leave them with large amounts of cash in rural areas where there were more bandits than police.[9]

The international scientific community, at least initially, was not enthusiastic. In fact, there were "shouting matches" in meetings with several Diarrhea Center staff (personal communications, Richard A. Cash, February 5, 2005; A. M. R. Chowdhury, March 3, 2012). BRAC was talking about training 65,000 women with a protocol that had a 90% success rate. That meant that some women would make a solution too high in salt and their children would be at risk of dying of hypernatremia. The humanitarian mandate to "Do something!" was in conflict with the basic medical mandate "Do no harm." However, BRAC and the Diarrhea Center staff eventually agreed that fewer children were likely to die of hypernatremia than were certain to die from untreated diarrheal diseases; the absence of alternatives in much of rural Bangladesh was the deciding factor. The Diarrhea Center therefore continued to support BRAC's work and helped to collect and analyze the data that would eventually confirm the soundness of the approach (Bhatia, Cash, & Cornaz, 1983).

The scientists at the Diarrhea Center regarded BRAC's systematic, trial-and-error approach as normal science, appropriate for refining an intervention or theory until such time that the relationships between all key variables are clearly specified and a controlled experiment can be designed. Abed's charismatic leadership, his friendships with Cholera Lab/Diarrhea Center staff, and the Center's familiarity with BRAC's earlier health programs all contributed to a collaborative, research-based approach.

> The Cholera Laboratory was a science organization. They had created oral rehydration therapy by 1968, but in 1979, 11 years later, Bangladeshis still knew nothing about it, and the newspapers were asking why the Cholera Laboratory had achieved so little. When we started experimenting with ORT, the Cholera Laboratory loved it . . . at last their science was going to the people. They loved our work and we exploited their science. (F. H. Abed, quoted in Smillie, 2009, p. 254)

BRAC recruited Oral Rehydration Workers (ORWs, Rehydration Workers) from among women living in the areas targeted for the program. BRAC advertised in a weekly district newspaper for women with secondary education and interviewed 40 candidates in 3 places, settling on 20. These Rehydration Workers then received 5 days of initial training, and groups of three or four of them were assigned to work out of one of BRAC's six camps.[10] After 9,000 women had been taught in Sulla, a new arrangement had to be created for areas where there were no BRAC camps. An independent team of 15 or 16 Rehydration Workers, headed by a male Program Organizer (PO) and assigned a cook, would make a temporary camp. Six days a week the Rehydration Workers visited one or more villages near this camp, chaperoned by the male worker. They traveled by boat and on foot, each Rehydration Worker training about 10 women per day. Every night the Rehydration Workers held a feedback meeting for 2 to 3 hours to discuss problems encountered and how they might be addressed. Finally, each worker wrote out 10 copies of the "10 Points to Remember" before bed because there were no printers in the field and during the pilot project, the message changed frequently.

At monthly meetings in Sulla, successes and problems were discussed. For example, some villages were confusing the Rehydration Workers with unpopular family planning workers and with disreputable women associated with traveling theater troupes already at work in the target areas. To counteract this, the male worker began to visit a village the day before the Rehydration Workers arrived to explain the purpose of their visit, particularly to elites. Some mothers were afraid that the *lobon-gur* solution would make them sterile, so Rehydration Workers began taking a sip of the solution in front of the mother. The monitoring found that some women were mixing two pinches of *lobon* and one "scoop" of *gur* instead of one and two, respectively, so the measurement was changed to one pinch of *lobon* and one "fistful" of *gur* to one-half *seer* of water.

To keep the program focused on effective learning, not just on the number of women trained, BRAC introduced an incentive system for the Rehydration Workers. A monitor would visit 10% of the women taught in the last month. The Rehydration Worker who trained them would receive a bonus for each woman who could make an effective *lobon-gur* solution, and then additional bonuses based on the number of messages the woman could recall. The incentive system motivated a new round of improvements in teaching methods. Before the incentives, for example, the Rehydration Workers simply demonstrated how to make the *lobon-gur* solution; now they insisted that the mothers make a batch themselves, in front of the Rehydration Workers.

As shown in Table 4.1, even something as basic as the number and content of "Points to Remember" was revised several times during OTP. Trial and error showed that 10 messages were too much for many mothers to remember, so several were combined. A message on the dangers of using too much salt in the solution was deleted, as the monitors learned that *lobon-gur* solution was underused (discussed below). As the number of households covered increased, BRAC learned that *gur* was not available in all villages, but refined sugar was, so the message again was changed, to allow equal amounts of either. As a result, the main training tool eventually became "7 Points to Remember."

One of the most fundamental changes to the "Points to Remember" came in the last year in OTP. All studies to that point had measured women's ability to make an effective solution; it never occurred to BRAC or its advisors that women might not be using it. However, the Technical Assistance Committee for the follow-on project, the Oral Therapy Extension Programme (OTEP), was planning a longitudinal study on the impact of OTEP and requested a study of actual rates of usage of *lobon-gur* solution to provide a baseline. The study's findings shocked all involved; trained women were using *lobon-gur* solution in less than 10% of all diarrhea episodes. In response, BRAC launched further research, finding that the ORT message only used one word for diarrhea—the one associated with severe watery diarrhea, the one most likely to be cholera. The usage rate for that type of diarrhea was much higher than for other types of diarrhea. As shown in Table 4.1, the final "7 Points to Remember" incorporated the four most common words for diarrhea, and by 1984, results of the longitudinal study found *lobon-gur* solution usage rates of 50% in cases of severe watery diarrhea and 33%, 12%, and 5% for the other three kinds.

ADAPTING NONFORMAL PRIMARY EDUCATION (NFPE):
LEARNING BY DOING

As was true for primary health care, primary education was not initially a top priority for BRAC group members. In the early 1980s, Abed and senior managers at BRAC expected that the government of Bangladesh would honor its commitments to universal primary education and would soon promulgate a compulsory primary education law. They further hoped that one or two cycles of compulsory primary education would eliminate the need for adult literacy and numeracy classes, if not for the critical consciousness components of BRAC's adult literacy programs. As a result, BRAC tried to frame its work in primary education, as in health, as facilitating access to routine government services for the children of the rural poor.

Background: Primary Education in Bangladesh

Before Independence, primary schools in Bangladesh were privately operated and served less than 60%[11] of children nationwide and a far smaller percentage of rural children. In 1973, the new government established its public education system by nationalizing about 36,000 privately owned primary schools. Government primary schools provided students with textbooks and approximately 157,000 teachers with salaries only slightly higher than those of a messenger in a government office (Government of Bangladesh, Directorate of Primary Education, Primary and Mass Education Division, 1999). Into the late 1990s, teachers' salaries consumed 90% or more of the government's primary education budget, and little funding went toward maintaining and supplying existing classrooms. Schools continued charging school fees to cover the cost of everything the government could not pay for: uniforms, textbooks when the government did not supply them on time, fees for taking tests, sports, and so on. Would-be teachers and their families pooled their resources to pay for a year's training at a primary teacher institute, and certified teachers struggled to survive on a salary that, meager to begin with, did not keep pace with inflation (Hossain, 1994).

In 1981 the World Bank and the government of Bangladesh launched the first of what became a series of large primary education projects[12] that initially focused on adding new classrooms to existing schools. Unfortunately, at the same time, lack of recurrent funds that meant many older classrooms were rapidly falling into disrepair, so the increase in classroom space was not even one to one. By 1984 only about 60% of Bangladeshi boys and 40% of girls of primary school age in rural areas ever enrolled in primary school, and far fewer completed the requisite 5 years. The reasons included

Table 4.1. BRAC's Oral Therapy Program, 1979–1987: Evolution of "Points to Remember"

"10 Points to Remember" (1979)	"7 Points to Remember" (Final version, ~1987)
1. Diarrhea is the condition of a patient who has more than one watery stool a day.	1. What are *dud haga* (diarrhea in breast-feeding infants), *ajirno* (indigestion from spoiled or simply too much food), *amash* (loose stools with mucous or blood), or *daeria,* (watery stool often associated with cholera) and their bad effects? These are all characterized by loose motions. With each loose motion, salt and water drain from the body. If this draining continues for some time, the body becomes dehydrated. Severe dehydration leads to death. So action should be taken to address *dud haga, ajirno, amasha, daeria,* or *cholera.*
	2. Symptoms of dehydration. The dehydrated patient develops certain signs and symptoms such as sunken eyes, dry tongue, thirst, sunken fontanel (in case of a child), severe weakness, reduced volume of urine, etc.
3. Treatment of diarrhea is oral replacement mixture, fluid, and food. 4. Oral replacement mixture is a mixture of sugar and salt in water. *Lobon-gur* mixture is one kind of oral replacement mixture. 6. You should begin giving *lobon-gur* mixture after the first watery stool.	3. Simple management of loose motions. The simple treatment for dehydration is to replace salt and water lost from the body. Remember, the patient dies of dehydration (loss of salt and water). So whenever a patient gets *dud haga, ajirno, amasha,* or *daeria,* give oral saline from the very onset of the disease (immediately after the first loose stool).
5. *Lobon-gur* mixture is made by mixing a three-finger pinch of salt (exactly up to the first crease of the index finger) to two-finger scoops of *gur* in one-half *seer* of tubewell or boiled water and stirring.	4. Preparation of oral saline. Oral saline is prepared with a three-finger pinch of salt and one fistful of *gur* in one-half *seer* of drinking water, well stirred. Care should be taken to mix *lobon,* water, and *gur* in the right proportions. A fistful of sugar can be used if *gur* is not available
7. For children, the amount of *lobon-gur* mixture should equal the water in the stools. If the mother does not know, let the	5. Administration of oral saline. Adult patients should take half a seer of oral saline after each loose motion. Children should be given only as much as they

Table 4.1. (continued)

"10 Points to Remember" (1979)	"7 Points to Remember" (Final version, ~1987)
child have as much as he desires. For adults, give one-half *seer* for each stool.	want, but at frequent intervals. Once saline is prepared, it may be kept four to six hours only.
10. Nutritional advice for patient with diarrhea includes: a. during diarrhea he should continue to take food and fluid; and b. after diarrhea he should take more than the normal amount of food for seven days.	6. Advice on nutrition. During *dud haga, ajirno, amasha,* or *daeria,* the patient should be given plenty of water and food like rice and curry, along with oral saline. In case of children, breast milk/ normal diet should continue. Increased amounts of food should be given for at least seven days after recovery. This will prevent malnutrition and weakness of the patient.
2. Transmission of diarrhea is by the anal-oral route. This means the feces of an infected person or a carrier enters someone else's mouth.	7. Prevention. To save ourselves from this illness, we should drink tubewell water. If unavailable, water should be boiled before use. Rotten food should never be eaten. All foodstuffs should be covered well so that flies cannot sit on them. Hands should be washed with soap or ash after defecation. Remember that breast milk is always good. Children put to breast immediately after birth and breastfed continuously rarely have *dud haga.*
8. *Lobon-gur* mixture can be dangerous when: a. too much salt is added to the mixture and b. infants and small children are not given small, frequent feedings.	None
9. A doctor should be consulted when: a. diarrhea lasts for more than two days, b. the patient cannot take fluid by mouth, c. the patient has severe diarrhea and cannot replace the water he loses in his stools with *lobon-gur* mixture.	None

distance to the school, fees for exams and uniforms, safety issues, and a curriculum irrelevant to rural life (UNICEF, 1987). In addition, schools were unfriendly places for first-generation learners[13]: many teachers were impatient when children had to be taught how to hold a book or a pencil, poor children were ashamed to go out of their neighborhood in their ragged clothes, and corporal punishment was common. Under these conditions, parents could see that their children were unmotivated and not learning enough to justify school fees or time away from useful work at home.

In the 1980s and 1990s, the World Bank, deeply invested in the notion of structural adjustment, required countries already deeply indebted to external lenders to adopt policies to make their economies more open to foreign trade and capital. It also required that those governments sharply reduce government expenditures on social services—like health and education—often by cutting or holding stable the number of civil servants, including teachers. Many large donors did not permit governments to use development aid for recurrent costs, such as teachers' salaries or teaching and learning materials. The Bangladesh government's ability to expand and upgrade the primary education system in the 1980s and the 1990s was therefore limited. At the same time, some smaller donors remained willing to fund all costs associated with humanitarian work, including primary education, in areas without access to government services, on a limited basis. It was in these humanitarian, stopgap terms that such donors began to fund nonformal education for children.

NFPE: South-South Exchange[14]

"Must our children grow into illiterate adults before they can join a BRAC group and learn to read and write?" BRAC staff say that this question from BRAC group members led them to begin experimenting with primary education as early as 1979.

In 1982, Abed gave responsibility for exploring better curricula for children's literacy instruction to Kaniz Fatema, a psychologist and social worker who had earlier joined BRAC as a materials developer for adult education. In 1981 she had participated in BRAC's 12-day training for adult "functional" education trainers and began thinking about how similarly brief training might work for primary education teachers. She visited a BRAC primary education school in Savar being run along conventional lines, which had dropout rates similar to those in formal schools. The school also lacked any form of community participation, an important element in most of BRAC's programs. She then began by making the rounds of the existing primary education institutions and projects in Dhaka,[15] including the Underprivileged Children's Education Program (UCEP, in Dhaka), a project in Noakhali funded by the Danish International Development Agency (DANIDA), and the National Curriculum and Textbook Board (NCTB). Initially she found nothing that seemed appropriate to the village context in rural Bangladesh, where few certified teachers were willing to work and where parents could not forgo children's labor for an entire day, every day.

Fatema's search led her to a small library in UNICEF's Dhaka office, where she found a brief report describing a project in Pune, India, that offered part-time primary school to children of the rural poor using paraprofessional teachers (Naik, 1980). Fatema shared the report with Abed, who suggested she visit Pune. There she saw village schools, attended training sessions, and interviewed staff at the Indian Institute of Education,[16] where the schools had been designed and were now being implemented as an action research project. Young women with 8 years of education were trained for a few weeks and then taught small classes of students in whatever space was available in their neighborhoods, including rooms in their own houses. The modular curriculum was organized on cards, each with its own learning objective, lesson, instructions for practice, and assessment. This plan covered 5 years of formal primary school in 3 years, allowing each child to advance at the child's own pace. The teachers and the children in the program all sat in a U-shape, on mats on the floor, as was traditional throughout South Asia. To Fatema these children's classes looked more like adult literacy classes than primary schools, but they seemed much better attuned to the rural context and to children's needs than did conventional primary schools in Bangladesh.

NFPE: The Field Experiment

The Pune approach seized both Fatema's and Abed's imaginations, but it took longer to persuade others in BRAC's education group of its value. Nonetheless, Fatema adopted only a few elements of the Pune model, which she began combining with prior ideas from the functional education training of trainers and her observations of BRAC's primary schools in Savar. For example, although the Pune model relied heavily on programmed learning[17] cards, she was convinced that children would prefer to have a book that they could hold, so she began writing the first primer, *Esho Pori*,[18] based on the books she had read to her own children.

Fatema arranged a workshop for a few BRAC staff beginning to think about children's education with Zahirunessa Syed, a U.K.-based education specialist. Syed helped BRAC staff to plan a curriculum for an 8-week preparatory phase at the beginning of the program, to introduce children without prior exposure to books and schooling to basic concepts about print and learning as a group. This preparatory phase had no textbook, only a teacher's manual. Syed also demonstrated how to use local materials—sticks and stones—and simple exercises to deliver a preschool curriculum.

Finally, in 1983 Abed requested that Fatema train the teachers in a new children's education pilot in Manikganj, close to Dhaka, where Fatema could keep a close eye on the results. Later she laughed about her early efforts:

> I didn't have the slightest idea how to train teachers, but I just took my *Esho Pori* and the cards. . . . [Remember] without [BRAC having] an education program I have developed these materials! [There was] no professionalism. . . . We didn't know [anything]. . . . Everything looks to me [now] like an accident. . . . [An assistant and I] took notes at a [workshop on preschool curriculum] and within a week we wrote that preparatory phase manual which has been used for the last 20 years. . . . We did not try out [before putting it into schools] because, [as] I told you, this was no frills. . . . (personal communication, Kaniz Fatema, December 20, 2006)

The lead-up to the launch of the new schools did not go smoothly. Fatema's supervisor and colleagues in the adult education unit were not supportive; they told Abed that children and their parents would not persist in a school with no books. Fatema said if they needed a book to show their parents, she would give them *Esho Pori*. At the first teacher training in 1983, most of the teachers were men whose schooling consisted of copying text into their notebooks; for them, even drawing a ball on the blackboard was a challenge. So she taught them orally and encouraged them to try out a wide range of activities. During this experimental phase, some classes, unable to find indoor classroom space, met under trees. Despite the skepticism of her colleagues, 6 weeks into the program Fatema found all the teachers and students—even those meeting under trees—"highly excited, 100% successful," carrying out a much wider range of activities, far more engaged than teachers and students in formal schools—and with no dropouts.

In mid-1984, BRAC established Nonformal Primary Education (NFPE) as a unit under its Rural Development Program, headed by Fatema and staffed with a field supervisor, a full-time education specialist, and several part-time curriculum developers. The first 3-year curriculum they developed included subjects considered relevant to rural children from disadvantaged families and within the capacities of some parateachers who had completed as few as 9 years of schooling: basic literacy, numeracy, and social studies/ life skills. A full 30 minutes per day were set aside for drawing, singing, dancing, physical exercise, and educational "excursions" around the village.

In addition, in 1984 foreign consultant Ignacia Mallon provided pro bono help with designing a 1-year stand-alone preprimary program.

Finally, the NFPE unit studied the funding proposal for BRAC's adult functional education program and developed one for a 3-year primary education program proposal for US$300,000. Without a precise measurement of the quality of schooling, something like the sodium chloride concentration test for *lobon-gur* solution, student and teacher persistence and parent enthusiasm became the most important indicators of educational quality.

NFPE Pilot: 1985–1988

BRAC's Nonformal Primary Education (NFPE) program was launched in April 1985 with 22 pilot schools in 3 localities where BRAC had other on-going programs and 1 where it had none, and grew to 787 schools within 3 years (Lovell & Fatema, 1989). During this time the basic features of NFPE's core school model were established, as shown in Table 4.2. The process of starting a school began, like much of BRAC's work, with a community survey by a Program Organizer (PO), the most junior of BRAC's staff members, who had received several weeks of training but was usually new to the rural area. Schools were established where BRAC found

- 30 or more 8- to 10-year-olds living within a 1-kilometer radius who had dropped out of or never attended conventional primary school;
- at least 70% of the out-of-school children were girls;
- several people, preferably young women, with at least 9 years of education, who were interested in part-time employment at market rates;
- parents would commit to sending their children to school for 2 to 3 hours per day, 6 days per week, 268 days per year for 3 years;
- the village was in close proximity to others with similar characteristics, making it possible for one PO to monitor 15 to 20 schools; and
- all villages were close to a BRAC field office where the PO would reside.

The PO worked with the parents to identify the most convenient school hours. In many communities, this meant that NFPE started in midmorning, allowing children to attend traditional early-morning religious classes. Vacations were brief and often planned to coincide with harvests or other times when children's help was most needed at home.

Once a decision was made to start a school, teachers received 15 days of residential training at the beginning of the 1st school year, weekly visits from BRAC POs, 1-day monthly refreshers at the local BRAC office, and

Table 4.2. Comparing BRAC's Oral Therapy and Nonformal Primary Education Pilots

Subsector	Primary Health	Primary Education
Program	Oral Therapy Program (OTP)	Nonformal Primary Education (NFPE)
Source of innovation	Oral Rehydration Solution Cholera Research Laboratory Dhaka, Bangladesh	• Adult functional education training of trainers, BRAC, Bangladesh • PROPEL, Institute of Education, Pune, India • Preparatory curriculum, United Kingdom
Target group	One woman/household	30–33 children/village
Deliverable	One 20–30 minute lesson	• 2-3 hours of lessons • 268+ days/year
Delivery cycle	2–4 weeks	2–3 years
Delivery agents	Oral Rehydration Workers • 8–10 years of formal education • 100% female Program Organizers (POs) • 12+ years of formal education • < 5 yrs of experience w/ BRAC • > 80% male None	Part-time parateachers • 9–12 years of formal education • > 80% female Program Organizers (POs) • 12+ years of formal education • < 5 years experience with BRAC • > 80% male School Management Committees (SMCs) Monthly parent meetings

several days of training before beginning Grade 2 and Grade 3. One teacher and one batch of students proceeded through the 3-year curriculum together in one room, all in the midst of a community that would closely monitor the attendance and behavior of both teacher and students. During the weekly visits, the PO observed the teacher teaching, checked the records, delivered supplies, followed up absences, held individual and group meetings with parents, and handled all school-related matters outside the classroom. A school management committee was also established and trained to help the PO monitor and keep the school running smoothly.

Table 4.2. (continued)

Subsector	Primary Health	Primary Education
Teaching and learning materials	• Posters • Gur (unrefined sugar) • "10 Points to Remember" • "7 Points to Remember"	• Blackboard, chalk • Charts • 1 slate/child • >= 3 textbooks/child/year • Writing and art materials • Teachers' guides • Record book
Infra-structure	• Umbrellas • Temporary lodgings	• Room >= 240 square feet • Mats (for sitting on the floor) • 1 stool for the teacher • Tin trunk for storage
Outcome indicator	• Chloride concentration test	• Attendance, persistence, satisfaction of students/teachers/parents, achievement on assessment-based on formal curriculum

In an effort to make the learning centers more self-sustaining, BRAC experimented with various levels of community participation, including very low levels of tuition, but as they had found with many health services, the amount their target group could afford to pay was not worth the cost of collecting it. Similarly, after several attempts to get the community to provide a classroom for the learning center, BRAC decided it was more cost-effective to rent a room. Over time, BRAC would conclude that parents needed to make just two contributions to NFPE: to release children from their chores for 2 to 3 hours daily and to send their children to school on time every day. Looking back, a senior BRAC manager who had been involved in earlier children's education efforts related the success of the NFPE compared to other BRAC experiments in primary education to one feature: "With Kaniz's program, everything is in our control: teachers, books, teacher training, buildings" (personal communication, M. Aminul Alam, January 28, 2007).

Like the oral therapy program, NFPE experimented and branched out in many ways throughout the life of the project. As early as 1987, in response to requests from adolescent girls, BRAC launched a 2-year Primary Education for Older Children (PEOC) program for 11- to 16-year-olds.[19] Also, to the surprise of all involved, more than 90% of the students who completed NFPE proceeded to join the nearest conventional formal primary school at the Grade 3 or 4 level. To better prepare the students to transition into the formal system, the NFPE curriculum was subsequently adapted to cover more of the formal primary school curriculum.

NFPE: Gender Issues

Girls made up a disproportionate number of out-of-school children in Bangladesh in the 1980s and 1990s. Parents were, with good reason, more reluctant to let girl children venture out of their communities to attend school,[20] and by the age of 6 or 8, girls provided valuable help to their mothers. Consequently, literacy levels among women in rural areas were much lower than for men. Locating schools inside the community addressed valid security concerns, as did keeping school hours short and selecting a trusted, respected woman from the community as parateacher.

Hiring women as teachers at the community level raised the status of women at the village level, provided role models for girls, and demonstrated to parents the value of girls' education. In strictly pragmatic terms, women with less professional preparation than men were often more open to adopting child-friendly approaches and less likely than men to move away from the community in search of better work elsewhere. In addition, there was little alternative employment for educated women in rural areas, so the going wage for part-time work was a small fraction of the already low wages of a government teacher. As with paraprofessionals in health, there was usually a surplus of candidates, and teachers who did not work out were quickly replaced. In the first 4 years, teacher dropout was only about 2%. In addition, of the 2% of teachers that became pregnant, most took unpaid leave and returned quickly to work. When they were sick, the teacher sent word to the school committee and a member or parent supervised class until the teacher returned.

For all its benefits, however, recruiting teachers from among women resident in the community where the school was located placed restrictions on how much training BRAC could provide. Initially, residential, preservice training was limited to 12 days, the limit most families said they could manage without mothers at home, even when trainees brought nursing infants to the training. Much inservice training and weekly PO visits to schools multiplied actual training contact time. Nonetheless, the decision to hire women teachers wherever possible meant that NFPE did not have the time to transform their candidates into the sort of activity-based teachers highly valued in the global North. By all accounts, however, BRAC teachers were more child-friendly and diligent in their teaching than better paid government teachers (Khan & Arefeen, 1992).

Although Kaniz Fatema, the director of the program, was a woman and the student body and the teacher pool were largely female, conditions of service resulted in field staff who, at least in the early days, were practically all male. POs were recruited at the national level, but were required to live in rural areas near their school with other BRAC staff; they were moved from one area to another based on the needs of the organization. POs were paid professional salaries lower than those obtained in the government civil service, but a growing program provided opportunities for moving up; almost all middle- and senior-level positions in NFPE were filled from within. As was the case with the teachers, the pool of candidates for POs was large and those who did not work out were easily replaced.

All of these employment conditions posed a major stumbling block for hiring female POs. Traditionally, young women in Bangladesh lived with their families until they were married, when they moved to their husband's household, often in another village. Married women stayed home to care for their household, moving only when their husbands moved. Few women rode bicycles or motorcycles in Bangladesh in the 1970s and 1980s, and those who did were often teased or worse. It was unacceptable for a young woman to be alone with men, so BRAC experimented with assigning female POs to team offices in groups of three. Still, the proportion of women in NFPE grew slowly. In later years, as BRAC instituted mandatory gender training for all staff, senior staff worked to make field offices more accommodating places for young women to live and work, but women still constituted a small fraction of the NFPE supervisory field staff for many years.

NFPE: Effective and Efficient?

For most of BRAC's staff, the program demonstrated its effectiveness in 95% attendance and completion rates for students, diligent teachers running their classes without corporal punishment, neater children eager to interact with adults, 80% attendance at parents' meetings, and happy parents. After the first 3 years, high transition rates—over 90%—to formal primary schools confirmed that NFPE was meeting the local standards of learning without the usual monetary or opportunity costs associated with after-school tutoring in formal schools. All of these features rendered NFPE a small miracle in the eyes of those familiar with the formal school system in rural areas, not to mention those who accepted the basket case label and judged Bangladesh an unlikely spot for an innovation. BRAC partially funded the NFPE field experiment and pilot with its own funds. In addition, Interpares (Canada) supported the 1985–88 pilot, joined by the Norwegian Agency for Development Cooperation in 1986, UNICEF in 1988, and the Swedish International Development Cooperation Agency (SIDA) in 1989

(Lovell & Fatema, 1989). The cost was extremely low per child, particularly for such a small program, because much of the support NFPE needed had already been established for BRAC's programs in other sectors.

Primary education, however, had no outcome measure as universally recognized and standardized as ORS had in the chloride concentration test. And as the number of schools increased, NFPE began to attract the curiosity of larger donors and of professional educators. In 1988, a World Bank–funded study conducted by education scholars at the University of Dhaka administered a test based on the government curriculum in mathematics, science, and Bangla to both BRAC and government students. The results showed,

> [Government] primary school students scored higher than BRAC students in all the [three] subjects. The difference of results of BRAC and primary school students in Bangla is minimum and not significant. (Begum, Akhter, & Rahman, 1988, p. 66)

In terms of cost, the report concluded,

> Per child cost in the BRAC schools is higher than in the government primary schools but if high wastage in the government schools are [sic] considered, per child cost of those schools stands much higher than the BRAC schools. . . . The World Bank has calculated that in a country like Bangladesh it takes approximately nine years of input (mainly teacher time) instead of the theoretical five years to produce one graduate of the primary system. Besides in the government primary schools, the teacher:student ratio is 1:51 . . . whereas in the BRAC primary schools it is 1:30. . . . The costs borne by the family for sending children to the NFPE centers are minimal. (pp. 68–69, 71)

The study did not make allowances for NFPE's abbreviated curriculum nor for the lower socioeconomic status—and therefore lower expected achievement—of its students. Nonetheless, the assessment was a wake-up call to BRAC staff: NFPE's successes, at least in part, needed to be measured in terms of learning.

Some of the report's recommendations, however, were inconsistent with conditions in rural Bangladesh in the late 1980s and early 1990s. For example,

> "All teachers should have at least 10 years of formal schooling."
> *Rural Conditions:* In 1988, sufficient female teacher candidates with those qualifications could not be found in many villages. Over time, as the government's female secondary scholarships and

stipends increased access to secondary schooling for rural girls, NFPE increased qualifications for teacher candidates.

"Extend the school cycle from three to five years."

Rural Conditions: The available parateacher candidates needed much supervision and many special teaching and learning materials just to teach Grades 1 to 3 well. Moreover, adding two more grades to each school would have increased cost, thereby reducing the number of children BRAC could reach.

As with *lobon-gur*, BRAC chose an essentially humanitarian approach, aiming to provide the maximum number of children with basic literacy and numeracy skills rather than providing more expensive, conventional primary education for fewer children.

CONCLUSIONS

Lobon-gur and NFPE were in the field experiment and pilot stages, respectively, when the world launched HFA and EFA in the late 1970s and late 1980s. The 1979 International Year of the Child inspired *lobon-gur*, but local demand—BRAC group members' request for children's literacy classes—prompted the NFPE experiment. As a result, the NFPE pilot had fewer connections to global goals and world culture than we will find in the next chapter. Nonetheless, both cases raise issues relevant to many of the single-country innovations that are so abundant in education and development case studies and perhaps also in international public health.

Both innovations described here emerged from an organization embedded in a context awash in pressing humanitarian need, among them high rates of infant deaths from diarrheal diseases and large cohorts of children quickly growing into a larger generation of illiterate young adults. Prior to the advent of the Internet, that embeddedness ensured that BRAC's innovations, although adapted from both national and international sources, could be somewhat particular to Bangladesh. The BRAC staff that initially undertook to adapt the Cholera Lab's oral rehydration solution and an amalgam of nonformal education models to the Bangladesh situation had no expert credentials in either primary health care or primary education. They drew on sector-specific experts at the Cholera Lab or from other organizations as the need arose. The lack of authoritative science undergirding BRAC's NFPE project raised few problems at the adaptation stage, but, as described in the next chapter, this lack became critical during scale-up.

Whether in health or education, adapting a promising innovation from one context to another involved much more than a quick tweak. Adapting the formulation of sterile ORS into homemade *lobon-gur* was by far the easiest part of the process. More challenging was

- identifying new types of delivery agents and adapting the deliverable to their capacities;
- developing support services based on the nature of the deliverable, the type of the delivery agent, and the location of the target communities; and
- determining how to maintain quality as the program scaled up.

All required substantial time and often several trials before achieving an acceptable outcome. Moreover, because the basic components of both innovations—a deliverable, a delivery agent, a delivery support system—were interdependent, a change in one usually necessitated a change in the others. BRAC, therefore, tested and adjusted each component multiple times in the course of field experiments and again during the pilot. Both OTP and, to a lesser extent, NFPE pushed past potentially crippling findings of low levels of effectiveness late in the pilot projects: the lack of effective use of *lobon-gur* and the relatively poor performance of NFPE (and government) students in mathematics and science. In both instances, BRAC revised its approach and resumed scaling up.

BRAC could use a trial-and-error approach to adapting both of these innovations in part because of the extremely low cost of conducting field experiments and pilots in rural Bangladesh. In most rural communities, BRAC found not just one literate woman ready to work part-time for modest remuneration as a paraprofessional, but several others ready to take her place if she did not perform. Having an executive director with private-sector acumen, one willing to put his own money into the organization, allowed BRAC to fund much of the adaptation process without having to prepare lengthy proposals for outside funders. External donors interested in population control, disaster relief for frequent natural disasters, and, increasingly, development provided a steady, relatively large stream of external funding to Bangladesh. However, programs able to demonstrate their effectiveness in empirical terms, governmental or nongovernmental, were scarce.

Of course, as summarized in Table 4.2 earlier in the chapter, in every phase and component, NFPE was more complex and costly than OTP. NFPE's delivery cycle lasted years, not weeks; the *lobon-gur* solution pilot took 1 year and NFPE's took 3. No single unit of instruction for NFPE— three-digit division, the past tense, personal pronouns—has ever had as much thought and research lavished on it as did that 20-minute *lobon-gur* lesson summarized in Table 4.1. OTP needed 2 weeks of logistical and pedagogical attention per community; NFPE needed 3 years. A couple of posters could keep Rehydration Workers going for hundreds of women, but thousands of NFPE students each needed at least three books and a slate. In terms of households reached, one Rehydration Worker served the same number in 3 days that NFPE teachers served in 3 years. Moreover, 2 weeks after OTP finished in an area, monitors gathered a few samples, conducted a quick chloride concentration test, and in less than a month objectively determined the effectiveness of the training. At this point in its development, NFPE had to depend on much less direct, interim measures of effectiveness, such as attendance and feedback from parents and teachers.

The iterative trial-and-error process of adaptation highlighted in these two case studies can be found in hundreds of other innovations for primary education and health in developing countries featured in anthologies and databases of education innovation. Precious few of these innovations, however, survived the field experiment and pilot stages; most succumbed to what development theorist Albert Hirschman (1975) called *fracaso*-mania or failure-mania: a tendency to declare failure too soon. In contrast, BRAC had experienced many "failures" from its earliest primary health and community organizing efforts and was prepared for a similar pattern in oral rehydration and primary education. And some donors, determined to provide support in an ongoing crisis where there were few other organizations— governmental or nongovernmental—with implementation capacity, tolerated more trial and error than they might have otherwise.

Hirschman also highlighted another pattern he saw in successful income-generating projects in Latin America in the 1980s, what he called "the first law of the conservation of social energy":

> Of the people principally involved [in successful projects], we found that most of them had previously participated in other, generally more "radical" *experiences of collective action that had generally not achieved their objective*, often because of official repression. (1984, pp. 42–43, emphasis added)

Indeed, quite a few of the early BRAC staff, including M. Aminul Alam, quoted earlier, had been members of the Communist Party as students, perhaps subject to some official repression, and Paulo Freire was indeed one of Abed's favorite theorists in the early years of BRAC. However, the parallel with Hirschman that we want to emphasize here is the importance of prior experience with collective action that failed. In our interviews, the founder of NFPE laughed about many things that had not initially worked out.

> I'm telling you about these incidents because these gave me an in-depth experience of what can work and what does not work. (personal communication, Kaniz Fatema, December 20, 2006)

She suggested that perceiving what will work and what will not is an implicit skill that she had learned, and could only learn, from trial and error and some tolerance for failure. As described in the next chapter, this is not a process confined to the field experiment and pilot stage; rather, it was BRAC's fundamental method for scaling up oral rehydration nationwide and nonformal primary education in a more limited way.

CHAPTER 5

Scaling Up

Blueprints, Bureaucrats, and Babies in the Bathwater

Colette Chabbott and Mushtaque Chowdhury

Small is beautiful but big is sometimes necessary.

—F. H. Abed, BRAC founder

In the annals of innovation and international development, the adaptations of *lobon-gur* and NFPE to the Bangladesh context have many parallels, but the speed and the quality of their scaling up have few. This chapter compares the factors at work in the nationwide scaling up of the simple health innovation and those in the later, less comprehensive scaling up of the more complex education innovation. In the discussion, we introduce three new *institutional* factors. First, in the decades following Bangladesh Independence in 1971, among development donors, development norms increasingly trumped humanitarian norms. Second, the development community struggles to construct activities where universal standards of quality are lacking. Third, the world model or blueprint for primary schooling—age-graded classrooms, professional teachers, universally appropriate for all children—is fundamental to the modern notion of the nation-state and as such resists innovation more successfully than does a much less powerful model for primary health care.

The reasons for the growing importance of institutional factors relate in part to the evolution of discourse about international development described in Chapter 2. Within the nation-states with the farthest to go to achieve the health and education MDGs, direct responsibility for achieving those goals lies, respectively, with ministries of health and education. For the most part, these ministries are organized along bureaucratic lines, often following colonial or more recent world polity models (Jang, 2000). The ministries often lack the expertise, the funds, and the implementation capacity necessary to realize global goals promptly.[1]

In the last half of the 1980s and into the 1990s, international development practitioners and academics broadly clustered under the heading of "development management" looked for ways to understand and reorient Third World bureaucracies toward better service delivery by increasing popular participation and accountability[2] (Bryant & White, 1982; Hirschmann, 1999; Korten, 1989; Lewis, 2007). In the process, several became intrigued with the potential of NGOs to expand alternative service delivery more quickly than governments could in underserved, usually rural areas of developing countries. Drawing on Argyris and Schön (1978), David Korten (1980) and Catherine Lovell (1992) specifically associated BRAC's ability to develop delivery systems in rural Bangladesh with its willingness to learn to be effective, to be efficient, and to scale-up, using trial and error to adjust to minor and major unanticipated issues *throughout the life of the project.* Korten and others (Brinkerhoff & Coston, 1999; Rondinelli, 1976) contrasted this learning approach with the blueprint approach more typical of bureaucratic organizations, such as government ministries and donor institutions.

The blueprint approach, of course, is never the *aim* of ministries or donor organizations. Rather, as in other organizational fields in the modern world, it is the predictable spread of standard operating procedures among international development organizations over time. For example, the use of logical or results-based frameworks at the project design stage—specifying inputs, outputs, outcomes, purposes, and goals, and associating them with objectively verifiable indicators and performance targets—began with the largest donor organizations. Resource dependence easily explains the spread of results-based frameworks to contractors and grantees of those organizations, but their adoption by NGOs all over the world may be better explained as a normative phenomenon, the result of the results-based framework coming to be seen as best practice. Subsequently, as the planners move on and implementation staff replace them, these frameworks often become institutionalized, and deviations from them come to be defined as failures in planning, implementation, or both (Korten, 1989). The blueprint approach thus privileges formal rationality over hands-on experience, and explicit over implicit knowledge. Moreover, the blueprint approach may encourage donors or bureaucrats to declare project failure too early, to throw the baby—the successful elements of the activity—out with the bathwater—the less successful elements—in other words, to succumb to the temptation to start over from scratch rather than learn the painful lessons at hand.[3] In the world of results-based frameworks, the temptation is particularly high for activities, such as primary education, that lack universal, quantitative indicators of cost-effectiveness or that challenge an institutionalized world model.

The notion that the details of an innovation can be resolved at the invention and pilot stage and that scale-up will require no further modification is not supported by either the *lobon-gur* or the NFPE cases described in this chapter. Rather, the trial-and-error approach of the field experiment and pilot phases continued in both throughout large-scale scaling up. The organizational and institutional environment in which this trial and error took place, however, presented fewer obstacles to *lobon-gur* than it did to NFPE. BRAC adapted and scaled up *lobon-gur* in a country less than a decade old, still recovering from multiple humanitarian disasters; with few government health services in rural areas; with the support of international scientists close at hand; backed by a global epistemic community; and under an authoritarian regime that gave NGOs a relatively free rein and government bureaucracies almost none. In contrast, when NFPE began to scale-up a few years later, development, not humanitarianism, was the norm among international donors, a shift that brought with it pressure to conform to global models of mass primary schooling, of sustainability, and of appropriate roles for government and NGOs. Moreover, NFPE had no international scientific community or scientists to back it up and later had to find ways to work with the first democratically elected national government, a government determined to redirect the flow of foreign funds for human services from NGOs to that government.

We analyze these two cases in chronological order, beginning with *lobon-gur,* followed by NFPE, using a five-part typology of scaling up derived from Korten (1980) and Uvin, Jain, & Brown, (2000):[4]

1. expanding number of beneficiaries/geographic coverage;
2. improving quality control;
3. diversifying core activities;
4. broadening direct and indirect influence; and
5. increasing organizational sustainability.

For the most part, we narrate the two cases separately and save systematic comparisons for the Conclusions.

THE ORAL THERAPY EDUCATION PROGRAM (OTEP): SCALING UP NATION-WIDE[5]

The oral rehydration pilot described in Figure 5.1 provided the basic operating approach for the Oral Therapy Extension Programme (OTEP). A Technical Assistance Committee that included the director of the International Center for Diarrheal Disease Research, Bangladesh (f. 1978, ICDDR,B, the

Diarrhea Center) as an *ex officio* member and other Diarrhea Center staff members guided many of the modifications described below. The committee was informed by studies undertaken by BRAC's Research and Evaluation Division (RED or BRAC's researchers), sometimes in collaboration with the Diarrhea Center.

Figure 5.1. OTEP: Basic Activities

The core activity of the Oral Therapy Extension Programme (OTEP) involved a female Oral Rehydration Worker (Rehydration Worker) going on foot, household to household in rural villages, teaching the "10 Points to Remember" to women one-on-one or in small groups in their homes. These points covered how to make *lobon-gur* solution with ingredients *available* in their village and when and how to use *lobon-gur* effectively. After a 20- to-30-minute training session, the Rehydration Worker made sure that the mother had understood the message by asking questions on each of the points. Most importantly, she had the mother make *lobon-gur* solution, and if the Rehydration Worker was not entirely satisfied with the level of understanding, she repeated the entire training session. Many Rehydration Workers took pride in their work, but all had an additional incentive to diligence; part of the Rehydration Workers' salaries were based on how many of their trainees could remember the 10 points when monitors came to test them weeks later.

One mobile team consisting of 14 to 16 female Rehydration Workers with a male cook and one male Program Organizer (PO) as team coordinator set up temporary quarters in an area. They followed a common "code of conduct," which stressed responsible behavior that adhered to local customs and culture. Men and women stayed in separate quarters, and no one was allowed to bring family members or stay with a family member. At 7:30 a.m., 6 days a week, all the Rehydration Workers made their way to the selected village and started working from different corners of the community. They tried to keep themselves as close to each other as possible in the village so that they knew each other's whereabouts. A Rehydration Worker's day in the field was over when she completed teaching 10 mothers. The team continued this protocol, day after day, for about 2 weeks or until they had trained women in 80% of households within walking distance of their temporary quarters.* Then the team moved to a new area and started again.

The team activity was suspended for 15 days every 3 months of work to allow the Rehydration Workers to return to their homes. During this period, the POs drew up field plans for the next 3 months, with guidance from their supervisors.

*Not all mothers were available during the Rehydration Worker's visit to the village. On average, Rehydration Workers were able to teach in about 80% of the village households during the pilot phase (Ellerbrock, 1981). Most of those not taught were absent from the house at the time that Rehydration Workers were teaching.

Source: Adapted from Chowdhury & Cash (1996, pp. 43–45).

Type 1 Scaling Up: Expanding Coverage and Size

As shown in Table 5.1, moving from the field experiment and oral therapy pilot described in the previous chapter, through the three phases of OTEP, cost less than US$1 million per year and took about 12 years. The program ultimately reached almost 12 million people, about 60% of all households, spread across 80% of Bangladesh's villages. During the life of the program, monitors interviewed 447,857 mothers and tested more than 330,000 samples of homemade *lobon-gur* solution. In the later phases, Rehydration Workers demonstrated the use of *lobon-gur* by treating some 427,000 diarrhea cases at the village level (Chowdhury & Cash, 1996).

Type 2 Scaling Up: Improving Quality Control

Korten, a frequent visitor to BRAC in the 1980s, argued that innovations are most effective at the field experiment stage; that in the effort to be more efficient (i.e., to reduce cost) at the pilot stage those innovations become somewhat less effective; and that efforts to maximize effectiveness and minimize cost (i.e., maximize cost-effectiveness) during scaling up will increase cost somewhat (Korten, 1980). Minimizing slippage in quality throughout these stages can help to maximize the number of beneficiaries effectively reached without necessarily increasing geographic coverage. BRAC's efforts to maintain and improve the quality of the work performed by far-flung Program Organizers (POs) and Oral Rehydration Workers (Rehydration

Table 5.1. Type 1 Scaling-Up: Expanding Coverage and Number of Beneficiaries; BRAC's Oral Rehydration Extension Programme (OTEP), 1979–1990

Phase	Years	# of trained households	US$ millions	Donors
Field experiment	1979 (3 mos)	245	??	BRAC (self-funded)
Pilot	1979–80	58,000	??	Oxfam, UK
Phase 1	1980–83	2,500,000	US$1.7m	SDC, Swedish Free Church Aid
Phase 2	1983–86	5,000,000	US$3.3m	SDC, SIDA
Phase 3	1986–90	4,300,000	US$4.3m	SDC, SIDA, UNICEF
TOTAL in Bangladesh	80% of villages	11,860,000 households	US$9.3m	

Sources: Chowdhury & Cash (1996), pp. 29–31, Table 3.1, pp 83–84, Table 4.1

Workers) led to significant changes in its oral rehydration program through-out the life of OTEP (see Table 5.1 for program phases). The program's con-tinuous monitoring system, developed during the earlier oral therapy pilot, formed the core of the quality control system, generating relatively quick feedback on the effectiveness of both technical and operational changes.

Longitudinal studies by BRAC researchers measured the longer-term impact of OTEP: how long women could remember how to make and use *lobon-gur*. In 1981 and 1984 retention among women trained in Phase 1 remained high for up to 6 months after training. The later study, however, also revealed that only 50% of women trained in Phase 2 could produce an effective solution and 25% produced a solution dangerously high in salt. Eventually, weak results were related to a shortage of mid-level field manag-ers at the peak of OTEP's expansion. BRAC undertook a variety of mea-sures to address this shortage, and by 1987 the 12-month retention rate for Phase 2 reached 90%. In 1993, 15 years after the pilot program, samples from all three phases found results similar to the 1984 study, with areas taught in Phases 1, 2, and 3 producing 71.2%, 64.4%, and 77.5% effective solutions, respectively.

Quality Control: Rehydration Workers. Because their salaries were based on how well mothers could make an effective *lobon-gur* solution, Rehydra-tion Workers were constantly on the alert for ways to reduce the margin of error in measurement. Based on their recommendations, confirmed as sound by the Diarrhea Center, the proportions of the formula were revised to make them easier to remember.

BRAC researchers found that teaching women in groups, rather than one at a time, reinforced the learning. Learning in groups also increased the likelihood that weeks or months later, when *lobon-gur* solution was most needed, someone in the neighborhood would remember how to make and when to use it. In Phase 3, therefore, the message delivery switched from individual mothers to groups of mothers and caretakers.

Quality Control: Monitoring the Monitors. Because money was involved and headquarters far away, monitors played a critical role in quality con-trol. They reported to senior managers, who scrutinized and adjusted the protocols that structured their work. Early in the program, for example, an unannounced visit found one monitoring team mixing *lobon-gur* solution, filling vials, and labeling them to send to the laboratory as samples from the field. After publicly suspending both monitors, BRAC developed a new protocol: Rehydration Workers recorded the name of the mother's young-est child during their visit and the monitor did the same when he collected solution. An Area Manager then confirmed that the solution came from an actual mother. Eventually BRAC's oral therapy program monitors themselves were monitored by BRAC monitors and both were monitored by both internal and external auditors.

As the expansion proceeded, the number of samples being collected for testing began to overwhelm the Diarrhea Center. Earlier it had determined that a simpler protocol for measuring chloride in *lobon-gur* solution could replace a more complex one without significant loss of accuracy. Diarrhea Center staff eventually helped BRAC establish a series of field laboratories, staffed by women with 12 or more years of schooling, to test the quality of the *lobon-gur* solution. To control the quality of the field labs, 10% of the samples tested there were retested at the Diarrhea Center, and the Center also conducted ad hoc spot-checks of the field labs.

Increasing Appropriate Use by Mothers. As noted in the preceding chapter, in the last year of its oral therapy pilot, BRAC researchers found that few women who knew how to make *lobon-gur* solution were actually using it. Besides changing the script followed by the Rehydration Workers, BRAC researchers began to develop new survey methods for monitoring behavioral change (Chowdhury & Faruk, 1982) and conducting qualitative studies of beliefs and practices about disease and treatment (Farazi, 1983).

Another reason for low usage was that *lobon-gur* solution was not a quick cure; vomiting and diarrhea often continued for many hours after treatment began. The longer these symptoms continued, the harder it was for mothers to believe that *lobon-gur* solution was working and to persist in coaxing their exhausted children to sip it. By setting up "clinics" where they treated diarrhea patients in full view of the community, OTEP workers were able to demonstrate the need for persistence in administering *lobon-gur*.

Type 3 Scaling Up: Diversifying Core Activities

In addition to replicating the same oral therapy program in more places, OTEP also added new activities and target groups for their oral rehydration message. For example, during the pilot phase, male POs had begun to visit elites in villages a few days before the Rehydration Workers began work, to explain their work and to help the village distinguish the Rehydration Workers from sometimes unpopular female family planning promoters. During BRAC's oral therapy program, POs also began to promote *lobon-gur* solution in the village where Rehydration Workers were working, meeting with men and boys in bazaars, mosques, tea shops, and schools. They also began holding village doctors' forums for physicians of all schools of medicine.[6] Finally, the Rehydration Workers also began setting up demonstration stations and treating cases of severe diarrhea in the villages themselves.

Type 4 Scaling Up: Broadening Direct and Indirect Impact

To manage the scale and scope of OTEP's communications activities, BRAC formed a new communications unit, which developed messages and media to promote *lobon-gur* in schools, on the radio and television, in public places, and with medical professionals and the government. As in all other areas of OTEP, the unit worked hard, but it had its share of failures. One example: restaurant owners, usually eager for colorful posters to decorate their establishments, firmly declined to display an anatomically correct poster depicting a patient in the throes of diarrhea. The poster was withdrawn. These communications efforts reinforced the message among those who had heard it, expanded the message to nonrural areas, increased discussions of the subject matter, and increased the authority of the message originally received face-to-face in an informal setting.

Finally, as noted in Chapter 4, in the medium term, BRAC decided that the best way to serve the largest number of the poorest people was to improve the effectiveness of government-run clinics in underserved areas. In late 1986 it began to facilitate other government efforts in child survival beyond oral rehydration, specifically providing child vaccinations and Vitamin A distribution in OTEP areas. BRAC's facilitation of the government health system went on to build on its comparative advantage in supporting delivery agents, often women resident in the target communities. For example, Bangladesh has a high tuberculosis rate, and treatment called for patients to take daily medication for 8 to 12 months. Compliance rates, as in many countries, were low. Beginning in 1984 BRAC sent *Shebikas* to directly observe TB patients taking their medication, and in succeeding years expanded and improved the protocol. In 1994 it began to partner with the government's tuberculosis control program. An analysis of performance between 1992 and 1995 in two of BRAC's subdistricts found the prevalence of tuberculosis to be half that of a comparison subdistrict served only by the government program (Chowdhury, Chowdhury, Islam, Islam, & Vaughan, 1997).

Type 5 Scaling Up: Increasing Organizational Sustainability

BRAC aimed to make teaching *lobon-gur* house-to-house unnecessary in a little over a decade. Its working hypothesis—that women trained by Rehydration Workers would train their children—appeared to be validated in studies of schoolchildren a decade after Phase 1 was complete. Indeed, ORS became widely available and used throughout Bangladesh by the mid-1990s.

OTEP increased BRAC's organizational sustainability in a number of ways. Many of the activities that BRAC developed to support OTEP—a research and evaluation group, staff training, a pool of female health workers eager to remain employed, personnel and payroll offices, a strong relationship with the Ministry of Health, and so forth—helped BRAC to expand other initiatives. These support services were established with some resources from foreign donors, but mainly with investments by BRAC from its own income generated by enterprises such as cold storage and the sale of program-support services, such as printing and the regional training centers, to other organizations.

Cost-Effectiveness and Impact

The impetus for BRAC's oral therapy program came from a desire to support the goal of the United Nation's International Year of the Child in 1979. While there is little doubt that BRAC's program contributed to this goal, measuring the program's exact contribution is not possible. As in many less industrialized countries, reliable birth and death statistics by age cohort were not available in Bangladesh in 1979 (or even much later). Consequently, individual Child Survival interventions in Bangladesh, including *lobon-gur* solution or Oral Rehydration Therapy (ORT), could not be measured against a reliable baseline. Further, during OTEP's later phases, the government began to manufacture and distribute ORS packets, complicating efforts to isolate BRAC's contribution. A 1993 study did show that using any kind of oral rehydration therapy (ORS packet, *lobon-gur* solution, or other homemade fluid) for all kinds of diarrhea had risen to more than 50% in areas covered by BRAC's oral therapy program 5, 8, and 12 years previously. For the most deadly type of diarrhea, the use rate was much higher, from 75.5% to 82.9% (Chowdhury, Karim, Cash, & Bhuiya, 1994; Chowdhury, Karim, Sarkar, Cash, & Bhuiya, et al., 1997).

Hard supportive data or not, internationally BRAC has been recognized for its important contribution to the reduction in fatal diarrhea. In 1992, UNICEF awarded Abed its highest honor, the Maurice Pate Award, for BRAC's work with *lobon-gur* solution. In 1994, a year after the 25th anniversary of the discovery of ORS, the Diarrhea Center recognized four agencies for their promotion of ORS worldwide: BRAC, UNICEF, UNDP, and USAID. About a decade later, the Diarrhea Center was the first recipient of the Gates Foundation-funded Global Health Award, and several years later, BRAC was the fourth awardee.

Winding Down OTEP

The difficulties of establishing the robust mortality statistics and thus the ultimate impact indicator for OTEP should be a cautionary tale to those donors who would demand measurable impact from national programs in less than 10 years. Even after investing in baseline and longitudinal data collection and analysis, the launch of the government's National Oral Rehydration Program (NORP) confounded BRAC's efforts to clearly identify the unique contribution of OTEP to Bangladesh's International Year of the Child or Child Survival efforts.

BRAC pushed hard to complete its oral therapy program in 10 or 11 years for several reasons. First, BRAC's working hypothesis was that mothers would pass on how to make and use *lobon-gur* solution—or, as they became available, ORS packets—to their children in the same way mothers passed on folk remedies. The government NORP program and the mass media campaigns it funded also helped to reinforce the message to a new generation. Ten years after the project ended, an education study of 2,100 11- and 12-year-olds found that over half of children with no education had knowledge of ORT as a treatment for diarrhea; of those with 3 years of education, 67% had that knowledge; and of those with 5 years of education, 79% had that knowledge (Chowdhury, Karim, Cash, & Bhuiya, 1994).

Second, BRAC wanted to complete the oral therapy program quickly because other development projects—such as primary education and village health workers—provided a better delivery method for simple, lifesaving treatments like oral rehydration therapy in a more sustainable way. As OTEP was winding down, BRAC was planning to scale-up NFPE to 100,000 schools, where making *lobon-gur* solution was part of the life skills curriculum, as described in the next section.

NFPE: SCALING UP . . . TO A POINT

Based on its experience with OTEP, BRAC conceived of nonformal primary education (NFPE) as another stopgap intervention that would be needed only for a few years, until the formal primary education system could expand into all rural areas. The rollout of the government's primary education system was, however, much slower than that of the public health system, and so NFPE was needed for a much longer time. Fortunately for BRAC, the project was successful beyond all expectations and by 1990 was singled out as one of a handful of particularly promising primary school innovations at the EFA World Conference. The two subsections below describe how BRAC increased NFPE from 787 schools to more than 11,000 schools in just 3 years, and the factors that subsequently led the organization to propose to scale-up in three phases to reach 100,000 schools by 1997. The number of NFPE schools, however, eventually leveled off at 32,000, as the plan for continued growth collided with both political and institutional brick walls.

NFPE Project (1988–1992)[7]

The design for the NFPE project built on the pilot described in the previous chapter, summarized in Figure 5.2, which provided 3 years of basic education for children who had dropped out of or never enrolled in school. Design issues and decisions were worked out in meetings with managers who had extensive field experience, though few had formal backgrounds in primary education. In addition, short-term international education experts sporadically advised BRAC on specific components of the program, such as mathematics curricula and gender. Program donors funded external project appraisals, monitoring reports, and evaluations every year or two, and these in turn informed program design. The program also grew some of its own expertise; for example, during Phase 1, NFPE sent 25 staff to the United Kingdom, the United States, and Thailand for certificates and master's degree programs in curriculum, education research, and other pertinent subjects.

NFPE's design and its implementation were informed as well by feedback from the field and by BRAC researchers. Initial efforts to hire a full-time education researcher within Bangladesh in the late 1980s produced no viable candidate, so BRAC sent several of its researchers to Canada and the United Kingdom for training. Initially, these newly trained education researchers focused on quantitative surveys and assessments in education similar to those they had carried out in health. Then they explored the larger context of education in rural Bangladesh prior to or while scaling up NFPE in some new areas[8] and assessed the performance of many NFPE graduates who went on to government schools.[9]

The sections below describe NFPE's scaling up using the same categories used above for OTEP: expanding coverage and size, improving quality, diversifying activities, expanding indirect influence, and improving sustainability.

Type 1 Scaling Up: Expanding Coverage and Size

As shown in Table 5.2, the number of NFPE schools grew most rapidly, by a factor of 14, during the first project. The largest number of these schools catered to rural Bengali children ages 8 to 11 years old who had dropped out of or never enrolled in conventional, formal primary school. The total number also included Primary Education for Older Children (mainly adolescent girls, f. 1987); the Education Support Program (described below, f. 1991); and a handful of schools for working children and children in slums (f. 1992). Throughout the scale-up, NFPE was known as a girls' education program, as it continued to enroll a higher proportion of girls than boys and to employ mainly women as teachers and men as POs.

Figure 5.2. NFPE: Basic Activities

A Program Organizer (PO) identifies 15 to 20 communities that are interested in starting NFPE classes, located close enough together to allow weekly monitoring by the PO. Within these communities, he or she identifies 30 to 33 children, aged 8 to 10 or 11 to 16, whose families own less than 0.2 hectares of land, who live within a 1-kilometer radius of the school, and who have dropped out of or never attended school, 60 to 70% of whom must be girls. If there are enough children who meet these criteria, two schools may be started in one community. If there are more children, a waiting list is maintained. The PO checks the list with the local government education officer to make sure that the students selected are not enrolled in formal school.

The PO recruits a teacher and a substitute from among married* women in that community or a nearby one with 9 or more years of schooling; if no women meet the qualification, a man may be recruited. The PO arranges for the teacher to attend 12 to 15 days of preservice training at the nearest BRAC Training and Resource Center. The PO then helps villagers identify or improve an existing space in the village for a classroom, usually a building with bamboo or mud walls and a thatched or tin roof, with a dirt floor and minimum floor space of 360 square feet. The PO assembles and brings all the teaching-learning materials to the schools, including textbooks and notebooks, a blackboard, a trunk, and a chair for the teacher (but no desk); parents usually provide mats to cover the floor. The PO then assembles the parents' group, securing pledges that they will send their children to school every day, on time, and that the parents will come to a monthly meeting. The parents help to establish the school timing and schedule. The school meets for 270 days per year, with brief vacations often timed to coincide with times when parents most need help from their children at home.

School meets for 3 or 4 hours per day, 6 days per week. The curriculum covers a somewhat abridged version of the formal school curriculum, using BRAC-developed textbooks, teacher's guides, workbooks, and activities. The curriculum has additional material considered particularly relevant to rural life. The first 8 weeks, the preparatory period, cover an abridged preschool curriculum: children are exposed to letters and stories; learn to arrange their learning materials and move into different-sized groups quickly; sing, dance, and play games; and form an emotional bond with their teacher. If students do not attend regularly during this period, others on the waiting list replace them. Each school day includes 40 minutes of singing, dancing, and games. If children are absent or not on time, the teacher and children may come looking for them. If the teacher is ill, a parent or the substitute may come to lead class. The PO may also follow up with parents of children who are late or absent during his/her weekly visit to the community.

Just before the school starts, the PO gives the teacher several days of preservice training, including lesson planning for the coming month. The PO then visits new teachers once or twice a week for the duration of the school and experienced teachers less often. S/he organizes and teaches the monthly refresher courses; keeps accounts of all materials; submits regular progress reports; participates in weekly team meetings; and, of course, maintains his/her motorcycle/bicycle. At the end of the cycle, s/he arranges for graduating students to enter the next level of schooling.

*Married women were preferred in order to reduce teacher turnover. Unmarried women were generally married in less than 3 years and moved to their husband's home, usually in another village.

Table 5.2. Type 1 Scaling Up: Expanding Coverage and Number of Beneficiaries: BRAC's Nonformal Primary Education Program (NFPE), 1982–2009

Phase	Years	# OF SCHOOLS Primary	# OF SCHOOLS Pre-primary	US$ millions (deflated[a])	External donors (from earliest to latest, * = also funded gov't)
Field Experiment	1982–1985	22	2[b]	<0.01 (0.02)	BRAC (self-funded)
NFPE pilot	1985–1988	779	0	0.3 (0.76)	Interpares
NFPE project	1988–1992	11,108	0	0.9 (1.54)	Interpares, NORAD, SIDA*, UNICEF*
NFPE 1	1993–1995	34,175	40	38.8 (55.64)	SIDA*, UNICEF*, NOVIB, ODA*, KfW*, DGIS, AKF[c]
NFPE 2	1996–1998	34,000[d]	1434	51.2 (66.40)	UNICEF*, NOVIB, ODA*, KfW*, DGIS, AKF/CIDA*, EC*
NFPE 3	1999–2004	31,183	16,019	128.5 (179.45)	UNICEF*, NOVIB, DfID*, KfW*, AKF/CIDA*, EC*
BEP 1[e]	2004–2009	33,250[f]	22,250[g]	188.0 (218.73)	NOVIB, DfID*, CIDA*, AusAID*, Royal Netherlands Embassy
TOTAL < 8% of national primary enrollment		179,527[h] 5.3 million[j]	129,986[i] 3.5 million	407.7 (522.24)	

Notes: a. OECD "Deflators for Resource Flows from DAC Donors (2009 = 100)," www.oecd.org/dataoecd/43/43/3498O655.xls; b. Converted to primary schools after one year (personal communication, Kaniz Fatema, January 8, 2012); c. As of 1993, NFPE donors formed a consortium that accepted a single common proposal, progress reports, evaluations, etc.; d. Excluding 517 hard-to-reach schools operating with no fixed cycle; e. In 2004, NFPE was rebranded the BRAC Education Program (BEP); f. Excluding 4,500 primary schools funded by European Community, outside of BEP Consortium; g. Excluding 4,100 preschools funded by UNICEF, outside of BEP Consortium; h. The number of classes exceeds the sum of one-room schools shown in this column because schools in some communities reopened for a second or third cycle. Also, in several phases, some schools operated on a 3-year and others on a 4-year cycle; i. Graduates and ongoing students in 2009. Until 2000, most graduates completed the equivalent of Grades 1 through 3; after that most completed the equivalent of Grades 1 through 5; j. In 2009 U.S. dollars.

Sources: NFPE & BRAC Annual & Progress Reports, various years; personal communication, Rubana Afroze, February 28, 2013; Ahmad and Haque (2010)

Initially NFPE scaled up in areas where BRAC had ongoing rural development or women's health activities, resulting in much better, more consistent delivery support than most formal schools in those areas enjoyed. In 1991, however, NFPE began working in areas outside BRAC's existing operations, somewhat independent of other BRAC programs, funded by a new NFPE donor consortium.[10] The project continued to draw on central BRAC resources, such as training centers, and also established other support services specific to NFPE, such as monitors. Having to start from scratch with communities meant that POs needed more time to read the internal dynamics—who were the leaders, what intracommunity conflicts might affect the school—and to establish trust. This placed middle managers, all of whom had worked as POs in more than one community, in a pivotal position, providing inexperienced POs with a second set of eyes and a larger repertoire of responses to community issues. Both in or out of BRAC's rural development areas, NFPE schools routinely received weekly or more frequent visits by POs, timely delivery of complete sets of teaching and learning materials, and school management committee training and regular meetings, resulting in high levels of teacher and student attendance and engagement.

Type 2 Scaling Up: Improving Quality Control

In comparison with most formal schools in rural areas, NFPE had more diligent teachers, better curricula, better support, and better parent engagement. These elements, in turn, produced higher attendance, more time on task in classrooms, lower dropout rates, more learning, and more completion, and increased the number of students for whom the program worked as designed. In the pilot and first project phases, NFPE teachers were called facilitators; classes met in temporary, rented centers; and the curriculum aimed to provide children of the rural poor with a self-contained basic education. In stark contrast to high dropout rates in formal schools, more than 90% of students completed the program. As described in Chapter 4, somewhat paradoxically, this success led 90% of NFPE graduates to enroll in nearby formal schools, most in Grade 4 (Lovell & Fatema, 1989).

Bowing to the wishes of parents and students, NFPE restructured its curriculum to better prepare children to persist in formal schools. Subsequently, BRAC researchers found that NFPE's simplified version of formal Grade 1 to 3 competencies did not handicap NFPE graduates when they transitioned into formal school (Khan & Chowdhury, 1991). NFPE graduates did, however, need more English—few NFPE teachers spoke more than a few phrases—as well as coaching to adjust to the lecture approach. Unfortunately, many of the same factors that initially discouraged NFPE students from enrolling in formal Grade 1 defeated them again in Grades 4 and 5:

crowded classrooms, rote learning, the time and cost associated with tutoring necessary for passing tests, distance to school and security issues along the way, clothing, and more (Mohsin, 1992).

The unanticipated desire of NFPE graduates to continue their educations and their difficulties in doing so resulted in the first of several shifts in the purposes—and the goal indicators—of NFPE. Over more than 25 years, NFPE's goal remained the same—to educate the children of the poor who had dropped out of or never enrolled in the formal system—but the terms by which program purpose and quality would be measured quickly escalated.

The NFPE field experiment and pilot had been guided mainly by qualitative indicators—parent satisfaction, teacher satisfaction, children's enthusiasm for school—and by close monitoring of attendance (by both teachers and students) and completion of the 2- or 3-year cycle. These indicators remained important through all phases, but during the NFPE project BRAC also began monitoring transition rates to formal primary school and the formal primary school completion rate for the 90+% of NFPE graduates who made that transition. Transition and completion, however, are output measures; they do not guarantee the quality of the learning outcome. Without a universal outcome measure, like chloride concentration for OTEP, or external sources to validate it, NFPE's measure of success was a moving target. As described below, BRAC's researchers led several efforts to develop valid quantitative learning assessments to measure the quality of NFPE and the mainstream schools in Bangladesh. These assessments largely established the relatively better quality of NFPE in comparison with formal rural primary schools, but it was not until the government established its own primary school completion exam in 2009 that the government began to pay attention.

Improving the Deliverable: Curriculum. Changing purposes demanded changes in the curriculum that, in turn, demanded revisions of textbooks and teacher manuals, as well as program organizer and teacher training materials. This was a far more arduous undertaking than revising the "10 Points to Remember" for OTEP. Improvements to the NFPE curriculum were constrained by the same factors that had constrained OTEP's much simpler "Points to Remember": time, pressure to keep costs low (to cover more children), and the limited technical capacity of the available delivery agents. They were also constrained by the size and complexity of the textbooks and the broad array of teaching and learning materials as well as PO and teacher training programs that had to align with those textbooks. Despite these constraints, the NFPE's teacher manual was revised five times during the pilot alone (Shordt, 1991, p. 353), an approach possible only for an organization that maintained its own printing press.

Improving Delivery Agents. In contrast with the oral rehydration program, NFPE was unable to devise performance incentives for its teachers and POs. Diligence on the part of most teachers was secured in other ways: the satisfaction many took in their work; lack of alternative paid employment for women; their increased status in their villages; close supervision by POs, school management committees, and parents; and the existence of other candidates eager to take their place.

A 1988 World Bank-funded study recommended that NFPE extend the preservice teacher education from 2 to 16 weeks, or a maximum of 124 days (Begum et al., 1988). As early as 1989, however, NFPE's training and PO visit system already provided its teachers about 54 days of pre- and inservice education and 100 to 250 on-site supervision visits over one 3-year cycle.[11]

NFPE's other delivery agents, POs, also needed a great deal of training. Often college-educated young men, few had experience with rural development or, in a highly gender-segregated society, working with women. One management expert described the role of these POs with approval (most likely to the horror of educators) as "similar to that of a foreman in a factory situation who closely supervised and guided each worker, i.e., teacher" (Jain, 1997). Although POs were expected to provide both administrative and pedagogical supervision, few were strong on the latter.

As the number of schools mounted, NFPE could no longer transfer enough POs and Team Leaders from other BRAC programs, so the program began to recruit and train new POs directly. All needed a battery of inservice courses, including BRAC's "effective supervision," NFPE's teacher training, BRAC's gender sensitization, and BRAC's training of trainers. During rapid scale-up, new POs often had to wait longer to attend these essential courses and, until then, relied on help from middle managers in the field. During periods of rapid scale-up, these middle managers, recruited from among the more effective POs, were often scarce. These middle managers were supervised by upper middle managers, who were supervised by regional managers. Eventually, in addition to being subject to BRAC's monitors and auditors, NFPE appointed some of its most experienced field staff as an internal monitoring unit, to provide quick responses to specific issues raised at meetings of regional managers in the field.

NFPE's needs far surpassed the level of logistics and support needed by OTEP. For example, the entire OTEP enterprise never needed more than a few vehicles and no permanent buildings. But to monitor 10 to 20 schools weekly for 3 years, each NFPE PO needed a bicycle or a motorcycle and a place to live full-time, within an hour or two's ride from the schools he or she monitored. While NFPE did not find ways to tie salaries to performance, allowing POs to buy their motorcycles in monthly installments provided a great incentive to use the motorcycles gently and maintain them regularly.

Maintaining Delivery Support. Most international management experts who observed NFPE came away impressed (Ahmed et al., 1993; Cummings, Dall, Fiske, & Al-Husainy, 1993; Gajanayake, 1992; Lovell, 1992). Monitoring and logistics—PO salaries, travel and transport, supervisors, logistics and management, lodging and offices, staff training—accounted for 39% of NFPE's budget. In contrast, teachers' salaries accounted for only 25% (compared with 90% in the formal system), teaching and learning materials 31%, and classroom rent and maintenance less than 5% (Lovell & Fatema, 1989).

Type 3 Scaling Up: Diversifying Activities

NFPE staff were encouraged to innovate and to look for ways the program might be improved or new activities might contribute to the greater goal. For example, the staff became concerned that many graduates of the adolescent schools were too old to continue in lower secondary school and, having no access to print materials, would soon lose their new literacy skills. NFPE organized some of these graduates into weekly reading clubs, supplying trunks stocked with mini-libraries and games. To further foster a learning environment in more villages, BRAC also experimented with village libraries, often located in formal secondary schools, and, in response to popular demand, established some adult literacy centers as well. Other new activities included a small scholarship program to help graduates continue in formal lower secondary school. NFPE also piloted home gardening centers on school property to help children and their parents improve nutrition within their limited means.

In addition to directly implementing new activities, by the beginning of the 1990s, BRAC began offering some NFPE support services to other, smaller NGOs. In 1991 NFPE launched the Education Support Program, which provided teacher training, textbooks, and PO training to other NGOs working in areas where BRAC had no operations. Under the supervision of an experienced senior NFPE manager, these schools eventually performed, on average, as well or better than those run directly by BRAC.

Type 4 Scaling Up: Broadening Indirect Impact

In 1990, 16 NGOs, which accounted for 90% of the nonformal education funding in Bangladesh, formed the Campaign for Mass and Primary Education (CAMPE, f. 1990) as an "NGO forum to network in the area of literacy and nonformal education," with Abed as its first chairman.[12] As one of its earliest activities, CAMPE helped launch a South Asia–wide communications initiative to promote girls' education. Using funds from

UNICEF and technical assistance from the U.S. animated cartoon company Hanna-Barbera, it developed a young female cartoon character, Meena. The campaign achieved high levels of recognition in participating countries (Communications Initiative, 1999). BRAC's leadership in Meena reflected OTEP's earlier learning about the value of social marketing in reinforcing messages among program participants and in extending those messages where NFPE was directly providing schooling.

Prompted by its successful partnership with the government on Child Survival, BRAC launched a Facilitation Assistance Program for Education (f. 1989, FAPE) with the Ministry of Education. The program worked with head teachers, school management committees, and parents to strengthen formal primary schools. According to BRAC's 1991 Annual Report, the program had covered 297 government schools out of 324 total in three *upazilas* (subdistricts) and showed "some modest improvements in some areas." An evaluation in 1992 was more candid: formal school teachers did not want to receive training or coaching from young men without the same or better qualifications. And without significant external funds for school improvement, most parents and school committees were not interested in being mobilized (Bangladesh Forum for Educational Development, 1992). Despite this "failure," pressures came from two directions to continue looking for ways to support formal schools. First, donors urged NFPE to continue trying to work with the government. Second, having seen how much collaboration with government could multiply the effects of current programs and increase long-term sustainability in health, BRAC leadership was determined to forge a relationship.

Together for Education?

At the 1990 EFA Conference, Barber Conable, president of the World Bank, hailed the BRAC school model as "brilliant," evocative of "a little red schoolhouse" (personal communication, Cole Dodge, February 14, 2007). And, indeed, the visual contrast between a conventional Bangladeshi three-room primary school and an NFPE school was dramatic. The conventional rural school was a brick structure with three classrooms filled with rows of dilapidated desks and benches, relatively bare of children's work. An NFPE school was a single room in an existing cane, mud, corrugated metal, and/or bamboo structure with a dirt floor covered with woven mats or burlap. The NFPE schools festooned their rafters and walls with children's artwork, and students greeted foreign visitors by singing "We Shall Overcome" in heavily accented English, but with gusto.

In September 1991, 18 months after the EFA conference in Jomtien, BRAC launched the *Together for Education* (1991, *Together*) initiative with much encouragement from UNICEF (Lovell & Fatema, 1989), BRAC's donor consortium (Shordt, 1991), and the World Bank. *Together* aimed to raise $270 million to open 100,000 NFPE one-room schools by 1997 and to provide 3 years of NFPE to more than 6 million children by 2000. At a time when formal primary schools were enrolling about 1.2 million students in five grades (Alam, Begum, & Raihan, 1997), NFPE proposed to deliver 600,000 students ready to start Grade 4 in the formal system at the beginning of the 1997 school year, increasing to 5 million for Grades 4 and 5 by 2000. The proposal framed this effort as "a major thrust towards implementing the government's [1990] Compulsory Primary Education Program" and as "a model of government-community-NGO partnership." The second point was particularly important because in order to absorb the additional students into Grades 4 and 5, the formal system would have to devote most of its existing and planned classrooms and teachers to those two grades only.

How does this radical scale-up compare with OTEP? OTEP's budget demanded a modicum of foreign funding and BRAC proposed the program at a time when the government's National Oral Rehydration Programme was in its earliest stages. In contrast, *Together* constituted an enormous request for foreign funding. More importantly, BRAC proposed *Together* after the government primary education system had already been in place for over 15 years. The World Bank had been channeling large but still woefully inadequate amounts of funds into that system for at least 10 years, and discussions were underway for a much larger multi-donor project. In those discussions the government's established, two-track strategy for expanding primary education simply did not include a track for mud-and-bamboo classrooms, primary schools of fewer than five grades, significant chunks of time for singing and dancing each day, parateachers, or a simplified curriculum adapted to be more relevant to rural areas.

Rather, the government's first track called for expanding the number of classrooms in existing government schools using its own and foreign donor funding.[13] With these new classrooms in place, the government then cut back school hours to accommodate two shifts per day in each school. In the second track, communities were encouraged to launch and support conventional secular and religious schools of three grades or more for at least 2 years, after which time the government would begin to subsidize 80% of teachers' salaries, with the intention of eventually nationalizing these community schools. A boom in these types of traditional private schools, largely staffed by untrained teachers, many with little teaching and learning material, today accounts for more than half of the increase in the number of government primary classrooms in Bangladesh since 1971. Schools in both tracks, however, received little on-site support,[14] and beyond a few favored schools, a highly bureaucratic system demoralized many teachers and their supervisors.[15] As enrollments in formal schools increased, so did the pupil-teacher ratio, reducing actual time available for instruction, further lowering the quality of formal primary education.[16]

As part of its efforts to persuade the government to adopt NFPE as a stopgap third track, in early 1992 BRAC's researchers developed and administered a brief achievement test to a sample of 11- and 12-year-olds in rural areas. Unlike the earlier World Bank–funded assessment (Begum et al., 1988), which aligned with the government curriculum, BRAC's Assessment of Basic Competencies (the ABC) measured "basic skills" as earlier described by the International Working Group on Education[17] and by international experts (Coombs, 1980). To increase external validity, an Interagency Committee including members from the government, Dhaka University, DANIDA, UNICEF, and the Diarrhea Center supervised the process. Using a 30-cluster sampling plan commonly used to measure immunization rates, the survey covered 2,100 children in 15 days for less than US$30,000.

The ABC's pattern of results diverged markedly from conventional examinations, which encouraged rote memorization. Boys who attended formal schools consistently performed better than girls on these examinations, and children from low-income households performed relatively poorly. In contrast, girls who had attended G1-G3 in NFPE, by definition from lower-income households, performed better on the ABC than any other group. Nonetheless, the proportion of students who passed all three subject tests was low[18] (Chowdhury, 1992). Similar to the discovery, on the eve of launching OTEP, that village women who had learned to make *lobon-gur* solution were not using it, the ABC found that 3 years of NFPE (or of formal school instruction) did not provide most rural children with durable basic literacy, numeracy, and life skills. The ABC findings suggested that despite relatively strong performance compared with formal schools, NFPE instruction needed to be improved and/or its duration extended. For the rest of the 1990s, BRAC's researchers continued refining the ABC and used it to track the performance of NFPE students, in some cases including comparisons with students from other types of schools as well, publishing their results in international education journals (Chowdhury, Choudhury, & Nath, 1999; Mohsin, Nath, & Chowdhury, 1994; Nath & Chowdhury, 1996; Nath, Khan, & Chowdhury, 1994; Nath, Mohsin, & Chowdhury, 1992).[19]

Meanwhile, international donor organizations continued to sponsor reports highlighting NFPE's technical and operational promise, among them USAID (Ahmed et al., 1993; Rahman Rahman Huq, 1992),[20] the BRAC Donor Consortium (Gajanayake, 1992), and UNICEF (Cummings et al., 1993). In November 1992, the Rockefeller Foundation featured

NFPE at a 3-day meeting on "Universal Primary Education in Bangladesh: Towards a New Vision" at its Bellagio Conference Center. At that meeting, BRAC had a place at the table with a former member of the Bangladesh National Planning Commission, who made strong statements in support of NFPE, and all present encouraged greater partnership between the government and BRAC.

NFPE Phase 1 (1993-1995)

During Phase 1 of its proposed scale-up, NFPE grew to 34,000 schools and then increased no further. The leveling-off appeared to have had little to do with the technical quality of NFPE or BRAC's capacity to expand and everything to do with changing relationships over time among government, NGOs, and elites in Bangladesh.

Government Pushback. The Bangladesh government had many good reasons for not partnering with BRAC to achieve compulsory primary education. First, a newly installed democratic government was determined to reclaim political space that the previous military government had ceded to donors and NGOs. International funding for primary education was on the rise, and the government was eager to ensure that as much of it as possible went into its newly created Primary and Mass Education Division.[21] Moved out of the Ministry of Education to be directly supervised by Prime Minister Begum Zia, the division was grossly underfunded. That some of the same donors who were funding recurring costs for NFPE, including teacher salaries, refused to fund the same line items in the government's primary education budget must have been particularly irksome.

A decade earlier, Dove had argued that, as in many other countries, "The obstacles to educational development in Bangladesh are not so much technical as primarily political" (1981, p. 165). She asserted that the 1973 government takeover of what were largely private primary schools was principally a strategy to make primary school teachers civil servants, thus coopting a highly politicized element at the grass roots. Without grassroots organizers, Dove suggested, the government would not be called to account for the limited progress in mass and primary education. Similarly, the announcement at the 1990 Jomtien conference by President H. M. Ershad, Bangladesh's military ruler, that primary education would henceforth be free and compulsory for all Bangladeshis was a grand political gesture leading to no new, financially viable initiatives.

In addition, NFPE impressed few government bureaucrats charged with planning and implementing primary education in Bangladesh. These bureaucrats had no formal expertise or training in primary education, so most did not recognize the technical merits of NFPE, nor were they interested in reading the dozens of studies produced by BRAC researchers described above. Government antipathy toward NGOs remained, and many dismissed the ABC exercise, designed and implemented as it was by BRAC researchers, as irretrievably biased, notwithstanding its international Interagency Committee. In addition, government officials who knew something about NFPE—for example, that the schools had no permanent buildings and devoted 30 to 40 minutes per day to song, dance, and games—dismissed them as "those song and dance" schools (personal communication, Erum Mariam, February 24, 2012). Furthermore, school buildings produce political capital for governments in a way that improving instruction does not.

Donor-commissioned studies of NFPE did not move most Bangladeshi politicians and government bureaucrats, since governments typically have little interest in research they have not commissioned.[22] They were justifiably skeptical of donors' passing enthusiasms regarding innovations in primary education. Programmed learning,[23] cluster schools, and satellite schools—some of which, like NFPE, used uncertified teachers and temporary classroom arrangements—had been or were in the process of being written into various donor agreements. None of these efforts recognized the importance of integrated support services, of incentives in ensuring high levels of diligence in the field, and of the quality of learning. Such officials argued that government and community schools could expand as quickly and perform as well as NFPE, given the same level of funding for both recurrent and development costs.

Finally, and perhaps most important, government documents from this period simply did not frame the lack of progress toward UPE as a crisis necessitating extraordinary, stopgap measures and partnerships with NGOs. Certainly the 4 years necessary to roll out its *National Plan of Action for EFA: 1991–2000* (1995) indicated a "progressive realization" approach to human rights described in Chapter 2. The plan, however, acknowledged for the first time that the formal system could not absorb large numbers of new students into Grade 4. The plan requested that NGOs already providing instruction in Grades 1 through 3 (mainly BRAC) expand their schools to Grades 4 and 5. Since BRAC had made it clear that the curriculum in those grades would be difficult for NFPE parateachers to teach well, the plan, intentionally or not, set up NFPE and other NGO schools for failure.

To respond to donor interest in NGOs, the government launched the Integrated Nonformal Education Program (1991–1996, INFEP, US$13m) without reference to BRAC's experience. INFEP included just US$5 million for children's education, spread among many small NGOs, many of them less diligent than BRAC (Ahmed et al., 1993). Later in the 1990s, the government converted a corrupt cash transfer program for the poor into a

Food for Education program in formal primary schools, targeting the poorest 40% of pupils. In 2000, grappling now with corruption in Food for Education, the government converted that program into easier-to-administer primary education stipends.[24] Both the food and the stipend programs had the advantage of increasing the apparent size of the government's education budget, moving enormous sums with minimal increases in delivery support, and appearing to target the rural poor. These programs were not principally designed to improve or reform primary education quality, and some question whether they even increased enrollments (Baulch, 2011).

Elite Pushback. In 1993 and 1994, elites in several areas of rural Bangladesh responded violently to BRAC's growing economic influence among the rural poor and, less directly, in rural politics. Attackers targeted BRAC offices and projects, burning 50 NFPE centers and forcing another 1,000 to close. BRAC researchers eventually identified three sources of the attacks (Mannan, Chowdhury, & Karim, 1994). First, at the highest level, religious elites knew that BRAC and other NGOs were largely funded by organizations associated with historically Christian countries and suspected that their ultimate aim was to disparage Islam and evangelize Muslims. Second, BRAC's work in various sectors threatened the status and livelihoods of several types of local elites, including moneylenders, faith healers, mullahs, and both formal and *madrassah* school teachers. Third, some new POs, most from urban areas, had not treated traditional religious leaders in rural communities with appropriate deference.

As had been the case with OTEP in Phase 2, these conflicts emerged at the peak of NFPE's expansion efforts, when the program was short of middle managers at the community level. Under pressure to start a fixed number of schools and without sufficient guidance from middle managers, a few inexperienced POs did not spend enough time in the target communities consulting elites and meeting with parents or simply did not recognize the gravity of preexisting conflicts (Rashid & Chowdhury, 1994). Following more intensive work with the communities, most of the closed schools were reinstated. Much as OTEP's Rehydration Workers integrated taking a sip of *lobon-gur* into their training protocol to demonstrate its safety,[25] NFPE demonstrated its respect for religion by distributing the standard religion textbooks used in formal schools to all its students, at its own expense.

The Donors Don't Deliver. Unlike BRAC's activities in most other sectors of its work, NFPE had no cost-recovery component; the program depended entirely on funding from BRAC's and donors' resources. Early in the field experiment phase, BRAC had concluded that the level of school fees that its target group could afford was not worth collecting. For an organization famous for recovering costs from that same target group for everything from chicken vaccinations to microloans, this was an astonishing but empirical conclusion. As a result, while BRAC enterprises generated sufficient funds to develop and test innovations on a small scale, large-scale continuation or expansion of NFPE required significant external funding.

Some of the international donors most able to provide the hundreds of millions of U.S. dollars requested in BRAC's *Together for Education* proposal, including the World Bank, however, were required to channel all their funds through government programs, such as INFEP. Other political and organizational factors helped to neutralize other donor efforts to establish a bigger role for NFPE in the national plan for compulsory primary education in Bangladesh. For example:

First, in the 1980s and 1990s, the World Bank's structural adjustment approach demanded that debtor countries slash their civil service and reduce social services in all sectors. Paying teachers, however nominally, was core to NFPE's success. Had the government integrated NFPE into its General Education Project, this largest of donors could not have agreed to pay the salaries of the parateachers and the POs.

Second, in the early 1990s, as development discourse reflected an increased interest in the role of NGOs in decentralized basic services delivery, it also expressed support for democracy and sustainability. If a democratically elected government did not want to work with NGOs, by what right could donors demand that they do so? Who better represented the will of local communities: local elites or a national NGO? If neither the government's nor BRAC's schools appeared likely to become self-sustaining anytime soon, did it not make more sense to invest in schools that were part of a permanent system, rather than in stopgap schools?

Third, in an organizational environment that prized universality and equity, NFPE raised the specter of the children of the rural poor sitting on mats in mud huts learning from their next-door neighbors, while better-off children sat at desks in brick classrooms learning from professional teachers. Thorny issues, such as different but equal (or better) types of education and trade-offs between learning and infrastructure, vexed many international development professionals and observers, as we shall see in the next two chapters.

Fourth, 2- to 3-year tours of duty in Dhaka for most donor and many government officials precluded developing and following a systematic strategy to build better cooperation between NGOs and government. The evaluation of NFPE Phase 1, for example, recommended that "to dispel [the] misunderstanding and mistrust" then characterizing government-NGO relations, an outside party should help with "goal clarification" and "conflict resolution" (Boeren, Latif, & Stromquist, 1995).

Fifth, donors pressed the scarce senior staff at NFPE headquarters to attend meeting after meeting to "coordinate" with government and donors, which they did, to little effect.

For these reasons, and likely others as well, the logic of supporting the government in its responsibility to educate all children in schools that conformed to the modern, age-graded, professionalized, Western model for compulsory mass children's education carried the day throughout the late 1990s and into the next decade. In contrast, the image of millions of children rapidly slipping into illiterate adulthood did not mobilize humanitarians the same way that child mortality had in health.

The leveling-off of NFPE expansion in the mid-1990s, therefore, did not reflect a technical limit on BRAC's capacity to manage more schools. Rather, it suggested the limits of technical arguments in introducing innovations in primary education. From a technical standpoint, NFPE as an innovation was

- adapted to the Bangladesh context by Bangladeshis,
- achieved similar or higher levels of learning than conventional schools,
- more effective for students not well-served by the conventional model,
- less expensive, and
- able to expand more quickly than the conventional primary school model.

For the rest of the 1990s and the subsequent decade, despite growing international recognition of the potential contribution of the NFPE model, the Bangladesh government effectively shut NFPE out of ever-larger donor-funded primary education projects. BRAC's 30,000-plus schools were not counted among those contributing to UPE in Bangladesh. For a less-established NGO with a less determined leader, this would have been devastating. Given the stage of development of NFPE and its scope, this was worse than throwing the baby out with the bathwater and more like throwing a teenager out of the family home. It was, however, by no means the end of NFPE.

NFPE Phases 2 (1996–1998) and 3 (1999–2004)

The government's disappointing response to the *Together* proposal strongly shaped NFPE's later phases. While it supported approximately the same number of primary schools, NFPE's budget in real dollars grew 20% between Phases 1 and 2 and 270% between Phases 2 and 3.

Much of the budget increase related to two ways NFPE expanded its schools without increasing their number, both of which raised the cost per student. The first type of expansion was a response to the EFA National Plan of Action; in 1997 NFPE began piloting Grade 4 and 5 and by 2000 most of NFPE's schools were covering most of the formal Grade 1 through 5 curricula. The second type of expansion came about as access to and incentives to attend formal schools, such as school feeding, grew in mainstream rural Bengali communities. In response, NFPE closed many of its schools in those communities and opened new ones in more marginalized communities, for ethnic minorities, slum dwellers, and working children. As described in Figure 5.3, these schools required further adaptation of the NFPE model, some new teaching and learning materials, and more intense supervision, all of which increased cost per child.

Figure 5.3. Adapting NFPE for Urban Contexts

In 1991, a field experiment in urban areas found that children there came to school with more exposure to print and shorter attention spans. They were rowdier and more aggressive (Khan & Khan, 1993). For example, most rural children need just one slate for their 3 years in NFPE, but in urban schools, slates were breaking right and left (personal communication, Saeeda Anis, 1992).

Teachers could not be recruited from the slum communities because most adults living there were fully employed, did not have adequate education, or moved residence too often. The middle-class teachers willing to work in the slums could not go there at night to find the parents of students who were tardy or absent. The curriculum developers had to add social studies units on kidnapping, begging, cleanliness, and skin disease. Parents who were suspicious of BRAC's motives took longer to organize. Initially, dropouts were high, some a result of bullying and others because young girls had many more employment opportunities in urban areas. NFPE's simple structure and lack of many of the outward symbols of a conventional school caused some parents social humiliation, and they withdrew their children (Khan & Khan, 1993). Early on, NFPE tried to establish the schools in the midst of squatter settlements, where the target group lived. The final report for Phase 1 explains that "school rooms have been used after hours for unsocial gambling, drinking, and have been vandalized in brawls between rival youth gangs"; therefore NFPE schools were moved to the safety of rental areas on slum fringes (BRAC NFPE, 1999). For all these reasons, urban schools demanded much more PO time and were more expensive.

The budget increases also reflected BRAC's diversification into three of the four types of scaling up discussed earlier, including broadening indirect impact, improving quality, diversifying activities, and fostering sustainability. This created scores of new stand-alone activities and more modest adjustments to ongoing activities; some of those that survived the pilot phase and were scaled up are listed in Table 5.3. Below we describe a few examples.

Type 4 Scaling Up: Further Broadening Indirect Impact[26]

In August 1996 BRAC redirected excess funds from NFPE Phase 1[27] into a national conference to promote UPE in Bangladesh and to spur action to achieve it (Jalaluddin & Chowdhury, 1997). Timed to coincide with the seating of a new government, Prime Minister Sheikh Hasina inaugurated the event, all former secretaries of education were invited, and more than 600 staff of the government, NGOs, academic institutions, international donors, and research centers, as well as teachers and social workers, attended the inaugural session in Dhaka.

Among many recommendations for improving quality, several speakers emphasized the need for better learning assessments.

> Both learning materials and teacher education must be designed to undertake continuous formative assessment. A national standardized system for assessing basic competencies of children should be introduced for monitoring and management at local and higher levels. This should be relatively simple and implemented through periodic sampling. (Jalaluddin & Chowdhury, 1997, p. xxix)

After a year without government response, CAMPE[28] raised funds and conducted a large-scale, nationally representative survey of primary school achievement, covering both NGO[29] and government primary schools, nonformal and formal. CAMPE aimed to produce a report that was impeccably technical, statistically rigorous, and above politics. A working group, modeled on the "sentinel" sites concept in health,[30] was assembled. It was led by the director of research at BRAC and included members from national research institutes, the Diarrhea Center, the University of Dhaka, and several NGOs. The group pushed ahead with a survey covering 42,548 households, 885 schools, and 3,360 11- and 12-year-old children in 312 villages in all 64 districts of Bangladesh. The survey included three instruments: a version of the Assessment of Basic Competencies, a household questionnaire, and a school-level checklist.

The resulting *Education Watch 1999* report from CAMPE found reason for some hope: increasing enrollments, especially for girls; an increasing completion rate; and higher participation rates for girls from poorer

Table 5.3. Additional Approaches to Scaling Up*: BRAC's Oral Rehydration Extension and Nonformal Primary Education Programs

	Oral Rehydration Extension	Nonformal Primary Education
3. Diversifying Core Activities		
New groups	Men, bystanders of all ages and genders, schoolchildren	Adolescents (BEOC); urban children, hard-to-reach/working children, ethnic indigenous children (EIC)
New activities	Treating diarrhea on site in villages during Rehydration Worker visits; libraries	Health and nutrition interventions: deworming, school gardens Tutoring support for secondary scholarship exam for preschool completers and NFPE pupils Adolescent Development Program for KK graduates: Clubs, job-related training, libraries
4. Broadening Indirect Impact		
Working with government	Participation in Child Survival Program Govt aligns ORS packet with OTEP standards	Facilitation Assistance Program in Education (FAPE, 1987–1993) Primary Initiative in Mainstreaming Education (PRIME, f. 2001–2003) Government Partnership Program (GPP, f. 2003): Support to formal primary schools, including preschools attached to primary schools, training for teachers and for SMCs
Working with NGOs	Training for private medical practitioners & professionals	Support other NGOs to run NFPE schools (ESP), community libraries, mobile libraries Secondary school support
Advocacy	Radio advertisements	CAMPE, *Meena, Education Watch*
5. Enhancing Sustainability		
Institutions	BRAC Research and Evaluation Division BRAC Regional Training Centers BRAC field offices (regional, divisional, team) BRAC Donor Liaison Office BRAC Human Resources Department BRAC Management Development Center BRAC Printer BRAC Motor Pool Public affairs and communication office	
	BRAC University School of Public Health	BRAC University Institute for Educational Development

*Typology: Uvin et al. (2000).

families. It also found some reasons for despair: less than a third of children left primary school with meaningful learning. The authors estimated that at the current rate of improvement in education, Bangladesh could not meet the goal of providing 80% of children with a meaningful basic education[31] until the year 2082 (Chowdhury & Nath, 1999). A year later, CAMPE conducted another, similar survey, this time with a new assessment aiming to reflect competencies in the formal curriculum[32] (Chowdhury, Choudhury, Nath, Ahmed, & Alam, 2001). The results for this test were worse than those for the ABC in 2000, but were consistent with recent externally administered assessments (Government of Bangladesh, Directorate of Primary Education, 2001; Greaney, Khandker, & Alam, 1999). These and later *Education Watch* findings generated many policy discussions and provided an impetus for several donor-funded projects, but as of 2006, the government strategy remained relatively unchanged, as did the slow pace of achieving universal primary school completion.

Type 2 Scaling Up: Improving Quality Directly

As they had in health, BRAC researchers provided grist for NFPE scaling up and quality improvement in the form of more than 160 reports. In addition, donors supported appraisal and monitoring missions and many consultant reports.

NFPE's goal escalated over time, from providing

a. a basic education adapted to rural areas *to*
b. the foundation necessary to complete the last 2 years of formal primary school *to*
c. an equivalent primary education of equal or better quality than the formal system.

Under the last iteration of the goal, NFPE developed new teacher's guides and training as well as PO manuals and training so that NFPE parateachers could teach a simplified version of Grades 4 and 5 and POs could manage them. At one point in the late 1990s, NFPE employed up to 25 full-time curriculum developers to keep the Grade 4 and 5 rollout on schedule (personal communication, Erum Mariam, February 22, 2005).

NFPE's notions of pedagogical quality did not always align with those of international education experts. Few NFPE parateachers or POs—and, by extension, their supervisors or support staff—had formal training in education or themselves had experienced anything but rote learning and lecture-style teaching, enforced with corporal punishment. To decorate classrooms with children's art; to smile and invite children to speak; to encourage them to play for a significant part of each school day; to refrain from striking out at them verbally or physically; to notice and seek out absent pupils with kindness; to give extra attention to slow learners and those with disabilities: all this was revolutionary pedagogy in rural areas of Bangladesh.[33] However, being more child-friendly and performing better than poorly performing formal schools was not enough for most Western education experts (Cummings et al., 1993; Moulton, Rawley, & Sedere, 2002; Sedere, 1995; Sweetser, 1999). Helping its teachers and staff integrate more progressive pedagogy at the classroom level proved an uphill battle until 2006. At that point, as international linguists were helping BRAC to develop teaching and learning materials for language-minority groups, NFPE curriculum developers began to see how more child-centered activities might improve language learning in the mainstream Bangla curriculum, as described more fully in Chapter 7.

Type 3 Scaling-Up: Diversifying Core Activities

In a program that valued innovation highly, many new activities were piloted, improved, and rejected or scaled up. For example,

- deworming for NFPE students;
- tutoring support for NFPE students ready to take the secondary school scholarship exam;
- training in job-related skills and some income-generating programs for members of adolescent clubs;
- operating 11 formal, graded primary schools in order to demonstrate NFPE's improved instruction methods in a conventional setting;
- creating mobile libraries on rickshaws;
- establishing community libraries and offering computer training in them;
- strengthening private[34] secondary schools where NFPE graduates continued their education, including teacher refresher courses for math and English, training for School Management Committees, and organizing students to make schools more hygienic and attractive;
- operating 16,019 feeder preprimary schools in the catchment areas of formal schools, and
- providing consultants to community schools programs in other countries.

Type 5 Scaling Up: Enhancing Sustainability

As noted, given its creativity in cost recovery in other sectors, if any NGO could find a way to help the poor pay for good-quality schools, it should have been BRAC. Instead, as had been the case in primary health care, BRAC learned that poor families in rural Bangladesh were not going to invest scarce resources to send all their children[35] to primary school until they were more economically secure. Until then, BRAC concluded, schools that aimed to enroll and ensure that all children regularly attended primary school would have to be absolutely free, near the home, and absolutely safe. Absent such schools, the government would have to offer financial incentives—food and stipends—to persuade poor parents to send children to existing formal schools. Neither government nor NFPE schools, therefore, had the means to become sustainable until first-generation learners became literate adults with more earning power and paying more taxes than their parents had and the government concurrently directed the additional tax revenue to primary education.

On a smaller scale, NFPE contributed to the sustainability of quality improvements in the primary education sector by increasing the number of Bangladeshis with training and field experience in primary education and in curriculum and materials development. Many of these moved to other, better-paying NGOs or international organizations after they were trained by BRAC, but they remained in Bangladesh. BRAC University's Institute of Educational Development (f. 2004, IED) also began offering master's degrees in Bangladesh in early childhood development and in educational leadership, policy, and management.

By the end of Phase 3, NFPE had adopted the formal school competencies as the framework for its primary curriculum, expanded most its schools to cover the full primary cycle, and saw most of its students' transition into formal secondary schools (Grades 6–10). In fact, not much "nonformal" was left in NFPE. In addition, work in other levels of education—preprimary schools, secondary schools, community libraries, and the like—meant that NFPE was no longer strictly a primary program. After Phase 3, therefore, BRAC rebranded NFPE as the BRAC Education Program (BEP) and expected the number of its primary schools to shrink dramatically. At least until 2013, however, many out-of-school children remained in hard-to-reach areas, and demand for NFPE schools remained high.

NFPE: Cost-Effectiveness and Impact

As shown in Table 5.2, the budget for NFPE (1989–2004), adjusted for inflation, was about $303 million. This is in the same range as the $362 million requested in the *Together for Education* to provide the first three grades of primary to all out-of-school children in Bangladesh by 2000, that is, in a little less than a decade.[36] In Phase 3 the length of the program expanded from 3 to 4 years, to enable schools to start and finish Grades 1 through 5 within the program cycle. Increasing training and field support for all delivery agents, diversifying into more remote and hard-to-reach groups, and adding more material-rich Grades 4 and 5 to most schools, accounted for much of the increase in average cost per student per year from US$18 (1985) to US$28 (2004).

In 1993, a small USAID-funded study in three subdistricts found that NFPE produced a Grade 3 completer for one-third of the cost of formal schools in rural areas (Ahmed et al., 1993). Further cost comparisons were not conducted until 2011, when BRAC funded a study of the economic and social returns of different types of primary schools in Bangladesh. Using *Education Watch* and household survey data, Ahmad and Haque (2011) estimated the completion rate for different types of primary schools and the private and social rates of returns of each type of primary school. Private, provider, and total costs for NFPE constituted, respectively, 29%, 78%, and 58% of those costs for government primary schools. With completion rates for formal schools at slightly above 76% and those for NFPE at more than 90%, Ahmad and Haque estimated that private and public returns on investments in NFPE were both about 3 percentage points higher than returns on investments in government primary schools.

In 2009, the government introduced a national primary school completion exam that permitted the comparison of the performance of several types of primary schools using an entirely governmental metric. Ahmad and Haque (2011) found that students who had participated in BRAC preprimary schools were more likely to pass the primary school completion exam than those who had not; the effect was especially strong among girls from poor families. This confirmed earlier sample-based studies conducted by BRAC researchers that found that NFPE female students performed better than their formal school counterparts in rural areas on both the ABC and the *Education Watch* assessment.

Finally, as was the case for OTEP and Child Survival, disentangling the impact of NFPE on UPE in Bangladesh is complicated by the rollout of three government programs during the same period that also aimed to increase primary enrollments: female secondary school stipends,[37] food for education, and primary school stipends.

CONCLUSIONS

International proponents of Child Survival and Universal Primary Education pointed to BRAC's oral therapy and nonformal primary education programs, respectively, to lend credence to claims that global goals could be met quickly and at a low cost per beneficiary. The OTEP case supports these claims; the NFPE case does so up to a point. The effects of sectoral factors identified at the adaptation phase—such as the simplicity of the innovation and the support of an international research center—gave OTEP an advantage over NFPE. Trial and error at the field level as well as systematic research guided both programs, but the research produced by BRAC researchers working with the Diarrhea Center for OTEP provided more external validity and a more universal outcome measure than BRAC researchers alone could produce for NFPE. NFPE, attempting to scale-up a decade after OTEP, also faced more difficult political and institutional environments than did OTEP.

Organizational factors highlighted at the adaptation stage—strong leadership on the part of F. H. Abed and of Kaniz Fatema, continual trial and error at the field level, rigorous studies by experienced researchers— also played a role in the scaling up stage of both innovations. In addition, at a critical point in scaling up, the quality of both OTEP and NFPE suffered for a period from a shortage of middle managers. Such managers had significant hands-on experience at the community level and from that experience had grown adept at improving through trial and error, knowing when to push a community and which communities to avoid. In addition, no matter how its "Points to Remember" were simplified and refined and Rehydration Worker training improved, the role of POs in OTEP grew rather than diminished over time. Similarly, no amount of curriculum reform or step-by-step teacher's manuals or parent mobilizing ever eliminated NFPE's need for capable POs. The importance of POs in both programs reinforces a mantra from earlier work in the agricultural sector: when dealing with paraprofessional delivery agents—whether model farmers, Rehydration Workers, or NFPE teachers—training without on-site follow-up—at the farm, in the home, in the classroom—does not work. However carefully NFPE developed training, ad hoc problems consistently arose at the field level that demanded the tacit knowledge of experienced managers. The many levels of managers, supervisors, monitors, and auditors that emerged from NFPE's trial-and-error approach to program development accounted for about 40% of NFPE's budget. This was a level that few development donors would accept from a government program, particularly in the 1990s when a central tenet of the World Bank's Structural Adjustment Programs was to reduce the number of civil servants.

In 1995, BRAC identified several organizational characteristics that contributed to the success of both innovations (BRAC Non-Formal Primary Education Programme, 1997; Chowdhury & Cash, 1996):

- prior experience in conducting development in rural areas;
- large, homogeneous context;
- management;

- planning;
- recruitment, training, and staff development;
- continuous innovation;
- staff commitment;
- communications;
- logistics;
- feedback; and
- coordination.

OTEP, however, had several features that NFPE lacked, including:

- international expertise playing an active role with the Technical Advisory Committee,
- support from an international research institute,
- funding readily available from internal and external sources,
- government support or at least nonresistance, and
- performance-based salary.

In turn, NFPE had at least one feature distinct from OTEP: the preexistence of many types of delivery support services.

Few government or nongovernment organizations in the countries with the farthest to go to achieve EFA enjoyed a similar constellation of organizational factors. Moreover, the time needed to adapt and pilot one simple health and one complex education innovation was, respectively, 1 and 6 years. OTEP took 10 years to reach 80% of villages and NFPE took 6 years (NFPE project plus NFPE Phase 1) to reach 10% to 20% of children in rural areas for a total of about US$9.3 million and US$58 million, respectively.[38] Both time frames exceeded the typical funding cycles for most international funding organizations. In addition, the trial-and-error process they both relied on has become increasingly unpopular, as standards for measurement, project design, implementation, and evaluation in funding organizations have become more rationalized and exacting.

In this chapter we also concluded that political factors played a role in the leveling-off of NFPE at well below national coverage. Dove, quoted earlier, argued that change could not come to rural areas without grassroots organizers. Twenty years after independence, BRAC and other NGO field staff indeed were ready to play that role and posed a threat to local elites. The ABC and *Education Watch* revealed weaknesses at the core of the primary education system, and to the extent that they acknowledged those weaknesses, government bureaucrats and politicians needed to demonstrate to donors that they were capable of addressing those weaknesses without the help of NGOs.

Finally, at least four institutional factors also prevented NFPE from scaling up as easily as OTEP had. Recalling our earlier definition, these factors define what is possible or legitimate in a given context and become so taken for granted that no special efforts on the part of individuals or organizations are required to keep them in place. First, the previous chapter described a self-directed NGO responding to rural problems in the 1970s and 1980s following a devastating conflict, in somewhat of a governmental vacuum. In the intervening decades, the Bangladesh government had acceded to a number of international declarations and agreements and had established a set of ministries consistent with world models. Each successive agreement was more effective than the previous at extracting national plans with specific, ambitious goals to which international donors attempted to hold national governments accountable, even as the donors were unwilling to fund them. Evidence mounted that the bureaucracy in Bangladesh was among the most dysfunctional (Asian Development Bank, 2007) and corrupt (Molla, 2005) in the world and that BRAC could scale-up an alternative, effective, accountable model without such problems. Donors, however, seemed to forget the eclectic mix of government and nongovernment models that had brought universal primary education to their own countries. Ultimately, by the early 1990s, both donors and government appeared to agree that primary education was a government responsibility and would be delivered through government channels.

Second, increasing tensions appear between Western humanitarian norms, shared equally among actors in the early decades of Bangladesh independence, and more rigid norms that subsequently crystalized in international development organizations. International development norms privilege a school system that aspires to be permanent, however weak, rather than a temporary stopgap, however pressing the need or effective the alternative model. No donors appeared prepared to acknowledge the length of time likely to be necessary to develop a universal permanent education system of reasonable quality and, by extension, to estimate the number of children who would go unreached in the interim. Even as the limited coverage and ineffective instruction of conventional primary schools were consigning millions of children to an illiterate adulthood, BRAC could not convince the government and donors that this constituted a humanitarian disaster, worthy of an alternative, temporary approach.

Third, OTEP's universal quality indicator—the chloride concentration test—was established early on and remained valid and acceptable to all parties at every phase of scaling up. Surveys established that trained women's use of the *lobon-gur* supplemented but did not replace the chloride concentration test. In contrast, NFPE's quality indicators were a moving target throughout all phases of the program: from satisfied parents, happy children, and high capture of a difficult target group (rural girls); to high levels of attendance, completion, and transition to formal upper primary or secondary schools; to progressive pedagogy; to high levels of achievement of formal competencies. As time passed, both donors and BRAC itself demanded more and more of NFPE. Direct comparisons with the nearest alternative—formal schools—were not possible until fairly late in the program, through *Education Watch*. The results of earlier comparisons of achievement favored NFPE, but the results were not conclusive for the government or some donors.

Finally, if our first point is correct, even had there been a universal, scientific quality indicator on NFPE's side, an international scientific community, or dozens of peer-reviewed articles in international journals, it is not clear that the government could have been persuaded to incorporate NFPE as a mainstream approach. The role of mass schooling in creating citizens for the modern nation-state means that control of schools will be much more contentious than the control of health clinics. To maintain their legitimacy, governments must effectively address epidemics, plagues, and natural disasters, but, crises aside, there are many models for primary health care delivery. In contrast, all bureaucrats have themselves advanced through formal schooling, know its uses and dangers, and, in the absence of other professional expertise, will want to follow a script consistent with the model they know best, especially if it has an international imprimatur.

Clearly two case studies in one country do not provide data sufficient to identify universal "lessons learned" for scaling up innovations in primary health and education. They do, however, suggest some characteristics of innovations, of organizations, and of contexts that may influence the speed at which innovations may scale-up and advance global and national goals, for good or ill, more quickly. Most of these will be quite unsurprising to those familiar with the management literature on innovation and theories of change, as follows:

I5.1.1. Tested and evaluated in a similar context,
I5.1.2. Piloted by delivery agents available in target context,
I5.1.3. Championed by at least one group with legitimacy in the
     international scientific community, and
I5.1.4. Rationalized in terms of quantitative outcome measures that
     have face validity with donors, politicians, and the target group.

In short, innovations do not spring forth fully realized, independent of their environment, whether organizational, cultural, or geographic. *Lobon-gur* and NFPE were the result of field experiments and pilots conducted in a particular context by an organization that was a product of and had experienced some earlier success—and plenty of failure—in that same context. This suggests:

O5.2. *An organization*—governmental or nongovernmental—has previously demonstrated its ability to deliver services effectively to the target context or a similar one.

O5.2.1. The organization has demonstrated its *capacity to learn by trial and error.*

O5.2.2. The organization has identified potential delivery agents in the target context.

O5.2.3. If it is not the implementer, the government supports the channeling of donor funds to an alternative implementer, such as an NGO.

O5.2.4. The donor tolerates trial and error well.

O5.2.4.1. The innovation can demonstrate effectiveness within the *funding cycle of the donor.*

BRAC had not yet demonstrated capacity to scale-up nationwide when it proposed OTEP. Therefore, again, the conditions described in these factors may not so much determine whether scaling up can occur, but rather how long it will take and with what degree of cost-effectiveness. The time factor in international development is a major one. Patient funders are usually small-scale; large-scale funders willing to wait more than 5 years to see reliable, cost-effective scaling up are rare.

Finally, contextual issues loom large, among them:

C5.3. The *size of the population* in the target context—an area unified by a common language, culture, livelihoods, and social structure—*justifies the cost* of initial adaptation, field trials, and pilots of the deliverable, delivery agents, and delivery support services.

C5.4. Within the target context, sufficient delivery sites are relatively *free from internal conflict.*

C5.5. A prior intervention has achieved similar levels and types of *community participation* within the target context.

C5.6. Delivery agent functions—e.g., teachers, POs, subdistrict and district supervisors—can be adapted to *labor available* at or willing to relocate to the delivery sites.

C5.6.1. An acceptable level of commitment and diligence on the part of delivery agents can be attained through some combination of salaries, performance incentives, and/or moral suasion.

In both cases, the large, dense, socially homogeneous population in Bangladesh justified the expense of program development, which focused on tailoring the deliverable to the available delivery agents, not the reverse. The issue was not simply how hard those agents could be motivated to work, but how much training and support could be provided to them in the target areas and whether this could consistently produce a deliverable of acceptable quality.

These contextual factors figure prominently in the next chapter, where Cholera Lab alumni and BRAC staff begin scaling out ORS and NFPE to other countries. Unlike Bangladesh, most modern nation-states comprise a plethora of contexts and lack a resident Cholera Lab or an Institute of Education, like the one in Pune, next door in India. The scaling out of ORS and of NFPE to other countries provided a natural test of many of the organizational, innovation, and contextual factors highlighted here. Not surprisingly, oral rehydration had an easier time of it than nonformal primary education.

CHAPTER 6

Scaling Out
From the Basket, Into the World

Other people in Goma used to laugh at us. "Oh, look at the people from Bangladesh! How can they help us when they have so many disasters themselves?"

A. K. Siddique, Head, Epidemic Control Preparedness Unit
Public Health Sciences Division, ICDDR,B (Siddique, 2003, p. 126)

The Cholera Lab's Oral Rehydration Therapy (ORT) and BRAC's Non-formal Primary Education (NFPE) began diffusing into new countries and contexts, or scaling out, as a response to global Child Survival and Universal Primary Education goals. In recent decades, international development discourse has increased its emphasis on the need for Third World countries to take "ownership" of projects funded by international donors. Support for such redirection, however, has been coupled with a reluctance to wait for homegrown innovations to emerge that can address the many critical issues confronting Third World nations. Many professionals working for international development organizations, responding to both humanitarian and development scripts, have undertaken to carry promising innovations from one country to another, in hopes these will jumpstart large-scale change.

It quickly becomes apparent in the two cases outlined in this chapter that scaling out into a new context may be no less time-consuming, resource-intensive, and trial-and-error-driven than was scaling up in the first context. Whether scaling up or scaling out, organizations must adapt and learn by trial and error, and some are better at this than others. Scaling out may require different delivery agents who need different types of deliverables and different types and amounts of support.

In this chapter, the speed of scaling out oral rehydration and nonformal education was constrained by many of the same sectoral, organizational, and institutional factors we identified at the end of Chapter 5. In addition, this chapter's cases present two very different ways of organizing scaling out, each with its own advantages and drawbacks. Oral rehydration therapy (ORT) scaled out in the 1970s, 1980s, and 1990s, led by international public health experts working with large budgets backed by at least one major bilateral donor. In contrast, when nonformal primary education (NFPE) scaled out in the 1990s and the following decade, its support came largely from UNICEF, a relatively small U.N. organization, working with the management-level staff of BRAC, a national (but soon the largest international) nongovernmental development organization based in the global South. In both cases it appears that the pace of scaling out was strongly influenced by the number of distinct contexts within a particular country and by the availability of organizations, governmental and nongovernmental, prepared to carry out program expansion by trial and error.

ORT: INTO THE WORLD

ORT's first venture into the world beyond the Cholera Lab was to India in 1971, where families in epidemic-wracked refugee camps near the Bangladesh border saved thousands of lives with it. The treatment spread rapidly, initially through individual scientists and then through organizations such as WHO. Improvement in communications was key to its diffusion. Eventually ORT became recognized as a cure for all diarrheal diseases, not just cholera, but its adoption outside emergency situations was slow.

The 1970s: Spreading the Gospel

> One Pakistani doctor, who was amazed to see the miraculous effect of ORS on one patient he was treating, [knelt] down by the patient's bedside, which was very dirty, and [said], "Allah, what have I seen?" (Barua, 2009, p. 82)

For many, regardless of their education or background, witnessing the "Lazarus effect" of ORT as it restores to life a child or adult wasted to a cadaverlike appearance by extreme dehydration is an eidetic experience. Many accounts describe the moment as seemingly miraculous. While BRAC was still learning to scale-up home-based oral rehydration in Bangladesh in the 1980s, dozens of expatriate alumni of the Cholera Research Laboratory (the Cholera Lab) in Dhaka and the John Hopkins International Center for Medical Research and Training in Calcutta (the Calcutta Center) had already begun diffusing the ORT gospel to other countries and to WHO, and finding uses for ORT beyond cholera.

Scientists as Carriers of Innovation. None of the international scientists associated with the Calcutta Center, the Cholera Lab, or, as it later became, the International Center for Diarrheal Disease Research, Bangladesh (f.

1978, ICDDR,B, the Diarrhea Center) were on permanent assignments. As research on ORT and on the elusive cholera vaccine continued at the Diarrhea Center, those involved in early ORT trials began to cycle out to prestigious institutions such as the U.S. Centers for Disease Control in Atlanta and the schools of public health at Johns Hopkins and Harvard universities. From their bases in these institutions, Cholera Lab/Diarrhea Center alumni applied for grants to continue research on ORT, which would bring them back, some for several years at a time, to Dhaka or to other parts of the world where cholera was still endemic.

For example, Norbert Hirschhorn, the researcher who had been surprised when doctors in Dhaka suggested there might be immediate use for his research (see Chapter 3), returned to Johns Hopkins University in 1968. In 1971, at the request of the U.S. National Institutes of Health, he conducted the first trial of ORT in the United States, on an Apache reservation. He was joined there by Richard Cash, who with David Nalin had carried out Hirschhorn's protocol demonstrating the effectiveness of ORT at Malumghat in Bangladesh. Their research on the reservation included not only microbiologic studies, but also *"the social and health system context in which health and illness occurred"* (Hirschhorn, 1990, my emphasis). Hirschhorn said the Apache study established three important points:

- ORT worked in young infants and toddlers with diarrhea caused by several kinds of microorganisms, not just in older patients with cholera.
- Infants drank as much ORT as needed for complete rehydration. They would then either fall asleep or cry for food.
- Early feeding did not make diarrhea worse, and ORT plus early feeding protected children from nutritional weight loss seen commonly with acute diarrhea (1990).

In 1975, Hirschhorn worked with WHO to design ORT trials in the Philippines and in the early 1980s led one of the largest of all ORT projects, in Egypt. The Egypt project included a massive social mobilization campaign that was informed by many ethnographic studies, which helped to establish the social and cultural features of the disease. By that time, Hirschhorn had cofounded a multidisciplinary private consulting firm named after John Snow, the founder of epidemiology, focusing on project implementation, training, and research in public health.

As for some other early ORT researchers (see Chapter 3), when politics in India led to the closing of the Calcutta Center in the 1970s, Dilip Mahalanabis (2009) joined the WHO Cholera Control team and worked with ORT in Afghanistan, Egypt, and Yemen. Bradley Sack went to work on cholera at the Naval Medical Research Unit in Peru, where cholera had returned after an absence of many years. Richard Cash went from the Cholera Hospital to the Harvard School of Public Health. He returned to Bangladesh and India many times to work with BRAC, eventually teaching in the James P. Grant School of Public Health at BRAC University (f. 2004). David Nalin went on to help establish a number of highly successful national ORT programs in Costa Rica, Jamaica, Jordan, and Pakistan. Jon Rohde joined the Rockefeller Foundation in Indonesia, and by 1974 an Indonesian organization had already begun manufacturing a double-ended plastic spoon that community health workers were teaching mothers to use in measuring a sugar-salt solution (SSS) at home. By 1978, the Indonesian Coordinating Board for Pediatric Gastroenterology was publishing research on ORT in its journal, comparing the double-spoon approach with other rehydration treatments (Sunoto, Budiarso, & Wiharta, 1983).

The World Health Organization Becomes a Carrier. The World Health Organization (WHO), the gatekeeper for many innovations in public health, did not immediately embrace ORT. Much credit for eventually winning over WHO goes to Dhiman Barua, a Bengali member of the WHO staff who in his East Pakistan childhood had seen his village doctor, the doctor's family, and many others die in a cholera epidemic for lack of intravenous saline. Barua's technical and professional credentials were impeccable: He studied medicine and bacteriology, and as a professor at the Calcutta School of Tropical Medicine, he collaborated on cholera research with scientists at the Calcutta Center (Barua, 2003a). His experience with managing cholera outbreaks was extensive; he spent a year with the WHO Cholera Control team in the Philippines and then, assigned to WHO's headquarters in Geneva, he helped pioneer the use of foil packets of the dry components of rehydration solution—waterproof and lightweight—in African cholera epidemics. In 1971, Barua traveled to the Bangladeshi refugee camps near Calcutta, where he witnessed Dilip Mahalanabis and a handful of Calcutta Center staff roll back a cholera epidemic with nothing more than sugar, salt, and a little bicarbonate. There, Barua (2009) said, the success of ORT under the worst possible conditions convinced him of its great potential in other emergency settings. The WHO team subsequently used ORT extensively in outbreaks of cholera among refugees during the Ethiopian famine in 1973–74 and again during the Bangladesh famine in 1974.

Many of Barua's colleagues at WHO were not as taken with ORT as he was. But Barua had eidetic experiences, technical authority, on-the-ground implementation experience, a growing pile of reports from international cholera researchers, and, finally, proximity to a key decisionmaker. His parking place at WHO headquarters in Geneva was next to Director-

General Mahler's. Eight years after the discovery of ORS, Barua finessed a chat that started in the parking lot into a 2-hour meeting with Mahler that

> put before him the favorable reports from the regions and countries of the role of ORT in the context of primary health care for one of the major killers of children, and also the resistance that was encountered from both within and outside of WHO. After very careful consideration, he [Mahler] advised me [Barua] to prepare a memorandum for his signature to the regional directors, along the lines we had discussed. This memorandum set the ball rolling to establish the WHO Program for the Control of Diarrheal Diseases (f. 1978, CDD). (2003b)

UNICEF and WHO eventually came to a joint agreement on a single formula for packaged ORS and issued guidelines recommending it for all types of diarrhea, for all ages, to be administered by anyone able to follow the packet directions.[1] Soon after the establishment of WHO's CDD, the formalization of international diarrheal control as a professional specialization began, and schools of international public health began offering courses in diarrheal diseases.

WHO's Control of Diarrheal Disease (CDD) Program. For at least its first 20 years, the focus of WHO's CDD program was ORT. Formalization, however, did not necessarily imply effective implementation. For example, Bangladesh, one of the first CDD-funded national oral rehydration projects to manufacture packets of oral rehydration salts in-country, mobilized its effort in part in reaction to BRAC's work to popularize *lobon-gur*. As often happened, though, the government lacked implementation capacity, especially in the rural areas where ORS was most needed. Therefore, the government program rolled out slowly. Worldwide, in addition to shortfalls in government implementation capacity, many members of the medical treatment community resisted administering ORT without medical supervision and resisted even more the notion of homemade ORS. In Cuba, for example, in the early 1980s, visiting public health experts were dismayed to learn that

> diarrhea in children, regardless of how mild, is always cause for professional intervention. At the first sign of "gastroenteritis," mothers are expected to take the child to the nearest polyclinic at once. Any child who has had diarrhea for two days is hospitalized. . . . To our surprise, however, we found no [instruction to mothers] about the importance of giving plenty of liquids in order to prevent dehydration. . . . "Definitely not," the doctor replied. "We don't want to tell the mothers anything that might lead them to put off getting adequate medical attention at once." (Werner, 1983, pp. 17–37)

ORT did not fit anyone's mental model of modern medicine. Families had been using less effective methods to treat diarrhea for generations and were reluctant to switch to something that seemed too simple to be true (Black, 1996). Even people bringing their sick to the Cholera Hospital in Dhaka would seek out family, friends, or any acquaintance at all on the Cholera Lab staff, pleading with them to order the nurse at the Cholera Hospital to give their exhausted, desperately ill relative some intravenous saline, not some silly sugar water (Wahed, 2003).

Within the international public health community, both proponents and detractors of ORT agreed that diarrheal disease was largely a by-product of poverty and unsanitary living conditions. Principally they were divided on tactics: proponents of primary health care argued that WHO's first priority should be directed to the source of all public health problems: poverty, manifested in crowded living conditions, contaminated water supplies, and poor sanitation. Prevention, they argued, was much more complex and expensive than using ORT to treat diarrheal disease (Klouda, 1983, 1993). In contrast, Barua noted that prevention proponents "had no recent advances in those areas to offer. . . . The Global and Regional Advisory Committees on Health Research kept advances on diarrheal diseases research high on their agenda for several years," and the area that was advancing the fastest was the use of ORT (Barua, 2003b, p. 138).

The Cholera Lab Becomes the Diarrhea Center. The United States had supported West Pakistan during Bangladesh's War of Independence. With Bangladesh no longer a member of SEATO and its new socialist government looking to the Soviet Union for help, First World security interest in the fledgling nation evaporated, and Cholera Lab support along with it. A network of Cholera Lab expatriate alumni, however, encouraged by the Rockefeller Foundation, undertook to broaden support for the Cholera Lab beyond SEATO countries in order to transform it into an international center, less dependent on U.S. aid. Several founders aspired to make it the first of several international health research centers focused on specific diseases located in areas where those diseases were endemic, along the lines of the International Rice Research Institute (f. 1960, IRRI) in the Philippines and the International Center for the Study of Corn and Wheat in Mexico (f. 1966, CIMMYT). With funding from Australian and British aid organizations, as well as USAID and WHO, the Cholera Lab eventually became the International Center for Diarrheal Disease Research, Bangladesh (ICDDR,B, the Diarrhea Center), and sent its first international epidemic response team to the Maldives that same year.

By 1982 WHO's CDD program was working with 52 countries to establish diarrheal control programs, and 30 were already manufacturing ORS packets (Centers for Disease Control and Prevention [U.S.], 1983, p. 1728). Some of these programs were more successful than others. For example, in some of the countries with very high rates of diarrheal disease, international agencies began to notice that ORS packets were gathering dust in warehouses, with few distribution channels and no demand from a population that did not know how to use them. In Pakistan, immunization teams left two free packets in each household, but when the immunization campaigns ended, so did the distribution system for ORS. In some countries in Africa, women were buying the sachets as a leavening agent for baking, because in humid climates, the bicarbonate[2] in the little foil packages stayed fresh longer than baking powder sold in the market. Just as BRAC had learned that mothers who learned how to make ORS might not remember what to use it for and how to administer it, demand for and use of ORS needed a boost, as described below.

The 1980s: Social Mobilization and Implementation

The Child Survival campaign was built around compelling summary statistics that spoke to political leaders and funders alike. In 1982, an alumnus of the Cholera Laboratory, Jon Rohde, argued that a few low-cost advances in medicine could eliminate half of the 17 million annual deaths among children in the developing world (Rohde, 1982). UNICEF's Grant (1987) argued that shrewd use of modern mass communications—radio, television, telephones—would greatly increase the number of people who could be mobilized in relatively short periods of time. Communication aimed at mass "social mobilization" leveraged UNICEF's limited funds and the much greater funds provided by other, larger donors, such as USAID.

Social Mobilization. In 1982, shortly after UNICEF declared it would focus on GOBI,[3] USAID chose ORT and immunization as its preferred approaches to health development (Northrup, 1993). USAID went on to sponsor three International Conferences on Oral Rehydration Therapy (ICORT, 1983, 1985, 1986) as one of its contributions to the global goals of the International Decade of Safe Water and Sanitation (1981–1990). Abed, BRAC's founder, was a featured speaker at the conferences, and BRAC's oral rehydration program was showcased. USAID followed up with funding for ORS production, distribution, and social marketing in dozens of countries.

Social mobilization could absorb serious amounts of funds. International for-profit and nonprofit firms, such as Hirschhorn's John Snow, Inc., and the U.S.-based Academy for Educational Development, responded and grew in this new niche for social marketing within the international development field. Some of these organizations piggybacked ORS campaigns on distribution and marketing channels already established for modern family planning methods. Elsewhere, ORT campaigns included large-scale surveys used to "segment" audiences by various characteristics, in order to tailor messages and distribution channels for each segment.

> In our research concerning the ORS product, we used sociologists, anthropologists, market researchers, clinical researchers and laboratories. We studied the attitudes, knowledge and practices of mothers, physicians, nurses, pharmacists, and the community in general. (Russell & Hirschhorn, 1987, pp. 237)

Diarrhea is not a subject of polite conversation in most countries, so selling a diarrhea cure requires a certain delicacy. Countries may comprise dozens of cultural contexts, and just as there were four words for diarrhea in rural Bangladesh, each context has its own euphemistic phrases and traditional treatments for diarrhea. Ideally, in each context and segments within those contexts, market researchers tested several media and messages for effectiveness.

In the short term at least, large-scale social marketing of ORS achieved remarkable levels of use. In Egypt at the end of a 5-year (1977–1982) national CDD effort by UNICEF and WHO, only 1.5% of mothers with children had ever heard of ORS, much less used it. By 1983, 2 years into an intense social marketing effort funded by USAID with technical assistance provided by Boston-based John Snow, Inc., one study concluded that over 90% of the population had heard of ORS and 50% of families with children under 5 years old had used it.

Implementation Takes Center Stage. Hirschhorn, chief of the technical assistance team in Egypt, attributed Egypt's achievement to assiduous attention to national leadership; to market research; to reconciling bureaucratic conflicts between the main funder, USAID, and the Egyptian Ministry of Health; and to developing three or more backup plans for every aspect (Russell & Hirschhorn, 1987). There was no blueprint for implementation. For each step, there were multiple backup plans, and many were used. Nothing goes as planned, Hirschhorn warned. The effort was expensive, but U.S. security interests were again at play. As part of the Camp David accords, the United States had promised Egypt large aid packages, and for projects with a scientific imprimatur, money was not an issue.

The factors contributing to the rapid scale-up of the Egypt project bore some resemblance to the list of factors at the end of Chapter 5. First, science was less pivotal a factor than implementation. As early as 1985, UNICEF convened a low-key meeting in New York with the following premise:

> The GOBI strategy is now enjoying widespread support. . . . *With the emphasis now almost entirely on implementation* . . . in an increasing number of countries . . . there is a danger that the program may promise more than can be delivered, and that enthusiasm and support may wane. (Cash et al., 1987, p. ix, emphasis added)

Diarrheal disease was among the leading causes of death for children under 5 years old in many countries. If ORT could effectively treat the vast majority of diarrhea episodes, a fully funded and comprehensive national ORT program might expect to halve diarrhea-related deaths in children under 5. Such dramatic numbers, over a million in some countries in 1 decade, played a major role in securing political will in international development agencies and among national leaders, and UNICEF's Grant, in particular, wielded the numbers with gusto.

At the time, however, many of the countries targeted for ORT lacked reliable records of births, much less reliable mortality rates disaggregated by age and cause. In Guatemala, some studies showed a drop in mortality of 55% following an effective ORT campaign. Hirschhorn (1987), more cautious, advised the UNICEF meeting that, given differences in implementation rigor in different contexts, a well-run ORT campaign could reasonably be expected to reduce overall child mortality by at least 9 to 15%.

Second, "implementation" was a catchall term for management, operations, logistics, and service delivery. Few countries had organizations, governmental or nongovernmental, able to reach remote areas and consistently train mothers to make an effective ORS with ingredients available in the home. As was the case with any national campaign, most countries had difficulty organizing and managing effective campaigns around ORS packets, not to mention sustaining their achievements. At meetings celebrating the 10th anniversary of Alma-Ata, several speakers, including Halfdan Mahler, focused on the lack of field-based, scientifically validated service delivery approaches.

> I would like to make a parting appeal to you that I consider it almost scandalous how little WHO has invested in research and development to try to support countries to find out how you really get optimal managerial approaches to delivering your meager resources. (Halfdan Mahler, quoted in World Health Organization, 1988, p. 100)

Third, momentum in a campaign is easier to sustain where there is a simple message and all involved stick to it. But research on ORT and implementation experience particular to certain countries did not stand still. Ongoing research on ORT was establishing that

- Mothers with several children and daily chores essential to the family's survival couldn't drop everything to administer ORS to one child until the child's diarrhea subsided, sometimes only after several days. It was essential to find treatments that would curtail vomiting and diarrhea more quickly.
- ORS given with food slowed down vomiting and diarrhea faster than ORS alone; therefore ORT should be defined as ORS plus food.
- Replacing the glucose (sugar) in ORS with cereal produced a formula that slowed down vomiting and diarrhea even faster than ORS and food.
- In countries that needed ORS most, a cereal-based formula was significantly more expensive than a sugar-based one. But cereal-based ORS looked a lot like the sort of foods, such as rice drinks and gruel, traditionally given to the sick. Over time, more attention turned to these foods, which were less likely to be dangerously high in salt than homemade sugar-based solutions and could be substituted where ORS packets were not available.
- Zinc could raise antibody resistance to future diarrheal disease.

Finally, the child saved from diarrhea today might, in a weakened state, be more vulnerable to and therefore die of another disease tomorrow. Conversely, a child weakened by a bout with malaria today might die of an otherwise treatable form of diarrhea tomorrow. Isolating the effects of an ORT campaign on the under-5-years-old mortality rate was difficult, if not impossible. Summarizing the findings of the 1985 UNICEF meeting described above, one commentator suggested that the Child Survival and Development strategies should be renamed the Integrated Child Survival and Development strategies, thus moving back toward a more comprehensive approach (Scrimshaw, 1987).

The 1990s and Later

Intense focus on GOBI interventions like ORT could not be maintained in perpetuity. In whatever time period they could hold the attention of major funders, Child Survival proponents hoped that a critical mass could adopt the GOBI technologies and provide a foundation upon which to build more primary health and development interventions. They were encouraged by the degree to which ORS distribution had indeed piggybacked on distribution channels for birth control pills and condoms. Child Survival critics, however, warned that, like most public health campaigns before it, short-term Child Survival would simply divert funds from the more important medium- to long-term investments in poverty reduction and from a more holistic primary health care system.

Both groups were right. Ten years after the 1985 conference, CDD was incorporated into the Integrated (read: comprehensive) Management of Childhood Illnesses approach. Attention to community-based services dropped dramatically, and by 2003 ORT was used only in around 20% of diarrheal episodes worldwide, although some countries maintained higher levels of use, including Bangladesh (Seidel, 2005, p. 62). Demand for funding for HIV/AIDS drew resources away from the Child Survival interventions, and within the Child Survival initiative, reaching the remaining pockets of polio that defied eradication continued to tie up funding and attention.

The need for ORT in emergency settings to prevent the spread of life-threatening diseases in the close quarters of refugee camps remained high. In 1984 the Diarrhea Center had created an Epidemic Control Preparedness Team composed mainly of Bangladeshis with extensive experience with cholera and other epidemics. The training team could rapidly deploy to countries with epidemics and coach medical teams on-site in effective management of cholera and other diarrheal disease.

ORT use in Africa was particularly tenuous. In 1994, the team responding to the Rwandan refugees in Goma, Zaïre, was disturbed by what they found and later reported in *The Lancet* (Siddique et al., 1995). Many of the health care providers they had come to train did not know basic protocols for rehydration or for appropriately identifying and treating different types of diarrhea. Worse yet, they would not consent to be trained.

The team leader recalled, "Other people in Goma used to laugh at us, 'Oh, look at the people from Bangladesh! How can they help us when they have so many disasters themselves?'" (Siddique, 2003, p. 126). Unable to teach, the team set up their own treatment center with the supplies they had brought for training. They improvised tents, hung IV sacks from nails on trees, cut used IV sacks in half for family members to use as cups for ORS, and gave mothers syringes without needles to administer ORS to babies. The team, per standard protocol, also set up a field lab and, as the cholera cases declined, determined what other strains of bacteria, besides cholera, were causing continuing high levels of diarrhea and which antibiotics were effective against it. The best antibiotic, they determined, was not the one the United Nations High Commissioner for Refugees (UNHCR) usually procured. Unlike many of the emergency medical staff at Goma, UNHCR was familiar with the Diarrhea Center's work and promptly procured large quantities of the antibiotic the team had identified, saving both lives and money (Siddique, 2003).

As 2010 approached, with the proliferation of discourse around capabilities and capacities in the international development field, combined with a surge of interest in "evidence-based policymaking" in the United States and other donor countries, the public health community was beginning to talk about "implementation science."

> We face a formidable gap between innovations in health (including vaccines, drugs, and strategies for care) and their delivery to communities in the developing world. As a result, nearly 14,000 people in sub-Saharan Africa and South Asia die daily from HIV, malaria, and diarrheal disease. . . . Many evidence-based innovations fail to produce results when transferred to communities in the global South, largely because their implementation is untested, unsuitable, or incomplete. (Madon, Hofman, Kupfer, & Glass, 2007, p. 1728)

Madon recommended replacing "trial-and-error optimization of health services, using descriptive studies, process evaluations, and monitoring to measure program outputs" with "implementation experiments—particularly cluster-randomized trials and agent-based models that compare the population health impacts of different delivery strategies" (p. 1729). But developing implementation approaches sufficiently well-defined and promising enough to warrant costly randomized trials should be the end product of many rounds of less formal trial and error.

In short, many factors accelerated the spread of interest in ORT to the world beyond Bangladesh in the 1980s. Most countries that adopted ORS took the packet rather than the homemade approach described in the previous chapter. As an intervention to promote child survival, ORT never attained the levels of coverage reached by immunization programs. Although not as complex as NFPE, ORT delivery was still much more complex than immunizations administered in a minute or two and demanding no one learn any new skills or undertake any behavior change. Moreover, ORT required a mother to decide several times a year throughout the lives of her several children whether an episode of diarrhea warranted ORS, whether to make or buy it, and how many hours to devote to administering it. Studies to improve implementation and to measure directly the impact of national ORT programs were surprisingly difficult to design and implement.

NFPE: SCALING OUT[4]

The ORT case provides one example of how an innovation can be scaled out when there are many enthusiastic innovators and early adopters, more than sufficient funds, and both donor and government engagement. In contrast, the NFPE case provides an example of how much more difficult it can be to scale out when there are fewer enthusiastic early adopters, not enough money, and limited donor and government engagement, a situation all too familiar in education in developing countries.

BRAC and UNICEF: The Big NGO and the Little IGO[5]

Although it dropped "Emergency" from its name in 1952 and branched out into many development activities, UNICEF continues to commit a substantial share of its resources to areas affected by disasters and conflicts. Given its relatively small budget and the high cost of international staff, UNICEF's ability to implement its own projects is limited. Instead, at least until the end of the 1990s, many of its field activities were implemented through local partners, including both national governments and local NGOs. In 1971, UNICEF joined a throng of disaster relief and development agencies looking for organizations that could deliver relief and development programs to devastated and remote areas of Bangladesh. Just a few years later it began funding BRAC.

In the 1980s and early 1990s, BRAC and UNICEF worked closely together. UNICEF executive director Grant's enthusiasm for BRAC's work was so intense that BRAC staff sometimes referred to him as "NFPE's grand ambassador" (personal communication, Kaniz Fatema, December 20, 2006). BRAC's founder, Fazle Hasan Abed, was chosen to receive UNICEF's prestigious Maurice Pate award in 1992 for BRAC's work in Child Survival. Manzoor Ahmed, UNICEF's most senior education officer, came from the same area of Bangladesh as Abed and had helped to include BRAC in a seminal anthology of rural development case studies (Ahmed, 1980). Moreover, UNICEF showcased BRAC's NFPE model in no less than three reports between 1988 and 1993 (Ahmed et al., 1993; Anderson, 1992; Lovell & Fatema, 1989). These three external reports, in addition to NFPE case studies in anthologies and other donor reports (Cummings et al., 1993; Little, Hoppers, & Gardner, 1994; Rugh & Bossert, 1998; Sweetser, 1999; Wolf, Kane, & Strickland, 1997), circulated among education experts working in international development organizations in Africa and elsewhere.

None of these reports or case studies or Grant's subsequent statements suggest that the BRAC model could be transferred more or less directly to another country. Ahmed et al. (1993), for example, highlighted several characteristics of the Bangladesh context that appeared critical to the success of NFPE, but might not pertain in other contexts, including:

- relative political stability,
- cultural and linguistic homogeneity,
- a large and capable NGO community,

- high levels of educated unemployment among women in rural areas, and
- dense populations in underserved areas.

The Ahmed et al. (1993) summary stated:

> Worldwide experience indicates repeatedly . . . that wholesale transplanting of an innovation from one country to another, without substantial "owner-ship" and sense of origination by the recipient country is "doomed" to failure. (Ahmed et al., 1993, p. 123)

The reports did, however, suggest that the model served as an inspiration and a proof of the concept that a poor country with a largely dysfunctional formal education system serving only a small fraction of school-age children could find a way to expand rapidly a low-cost form of primary schooling that was acceptable to local parents.

By the end of the 1980s, as BRAC's NFPE program scaled up and the notion of Bangladesh as an ongoing emergency began to recede, UNICEF encouraged BRAC to seek more funding from other development donors. By the end of the 1990s UNICEF/Bangladesh had become a minor funder for NFPE in Bangladesh. UNICEF headquarters, however, continued to promote BRAC's model as appropriate for South-South sharing well into the next decade.

NFPE: Varieties of Diffusion

In response to the studies and reports published about BRAC by donor organizations, hundreds of visitors traveled to Bangladesh to see BRAC's NFPE model firsthand. These study tours, in turn, prompted a series of pilot community school efforts in Africa and Asia, for some of which BRAC staff provided short- and long-term technical assistance.

Showing and Telling: International Visitors

Most of UNICEF's education staff in sub-Saharan Africa traveled to Bangladesh for exposure to the BRAC NFPE model in the 1990s and, in turn, sent many national delegations from African countries. Groups from China and Ethiopia visited on their own initiative, and BRAC accommodated many other unsponsored visitors at its own expense. Neither BRAC nor UNICEF maintained a comprehensive roster of NFPE's visitors. However, various NFPE reports included illustrative lists. The 1997 NFPE annual report, for example, mentioned visitors from Britain, Japan, Vietnam, Canada, India,

France, Pakistan, the United States, the Netherlands, Myanmar, Nepal, Bhutan, Iraq, China, Sudan, Uzbekistan, and Azerbaijan.

A former BRAC public affairs officer said his most difficult foreign delegation was a group of education ministers organized by the Association for Development of Education in Africa who came in 2003 or 2004. Several ministers expressed outrage at the lack of the most basic amenities associated with formal schools, such as ceiling fans, benches, tables, and latrines.

The ministers' insistence that BRAC meet "African" standards of acceptable infrastructure represents the reverse of a problem that several BRAC staff had already encountered in efforts to implement NFPE outside of Bangladesh: Some visitors were loath to change or adapt any aspect of the BRAC school model once they returned home. In Ethiopia, for example, BRAC staff noticed that the students were arranged in the traditional U-shape, around the perimeter of the classroom. However, instead of being curled up comfortably, the tall adolescent girls, unaccustomed to sitting on mats, had stretched their long legs stiffly out in front of them, taking up most of the space in a classroom sized to fit much shorter Bangladeshi children. When the BRAC consultant asked why the teacher didn't arrange the students or the classroom differently, the teacher explained that the BRAC model required that specific classroom size and seating arrangement.

Given the volume of visitors, surprisingly few returned home and attempted to launch readily recognizable NFPE-like one-room schools. Several BRAC staff members speculated that many visitors from the global South, both governmental and nongovernmental, perhaps found the scale and complexity of NFPE's management overwhelming. They suggested that some visits to BRAC's Education Support Program (ESP), which provided training, supervision, and curriculum development to smaller Bangladeshi NGOs, might have been more appropriate. This, however, begged the question of how small NGOs in other countries would have managed NFPE-like schools without the sort of support services that BRAC supplied to ESP schools, such as printing, curriculum development, and teacher training. In Mali, one of the best-documented examples of an attempt to adapt the BRAC model to another country without direct input from BRAC, an international NGO, Save the Children, played this role. The involvement of this Northern NGO dramatically raised the per-pupil cost of the model, but also enabled the Mali experiment to scale-up with more consistency and quality than any other NFPE model in Africa (Laugharn, 2001).

Sharing NFPE with the rest of the world, therefore, involved more than showing and telling and then encouraging visitors to go home and do likewise. Beginning in the early 1990s, BRAC senior staff served as short-term consultants to groups experimenting with NFPE in many countries. From the perspective of BRAC staff, these consultancies led, more often than not, to recommendations to do more trial and error and treat BRAC's NFPE as an exemplar, not a blueprint.

Coaching: Short-Term Consulting and Advising

Following the 1990 Jomtien conference, UNICEF invited the originators of both *Escuela Nueva* (EN) in Colombia and NFPE in Bangladesh to join the UNICEF education staff. The EN originator subsequently served for several years as UNICEF's Regional Adviser for Education in the Americas, where she helped promote adaptations of that model. The NFPE originator, however, agreed only to a handful of short consultancies in Africa and Asia. As had been the case with ORT at the Cholera Lab, donor and NGO professionals who had seen NFPE at work in Bangladesh played an important role in carrying its ideas elsewhere. One of the most active of these was Cole Dodge, the country director for UNICEF/Bangladesh in the early 1990s, who moved in the mid-1990s to become regional director of UNICEF's Eastern and Southern Africa Regional Office (ESARO). At the same time, Bangladeshi nationals working for UNICEF and other UNICEF staff who had previously worked in Bangladesh and were familiar with BRAC, served in key roles in Eastern and Southern Africa. One senior member of the BRAC NFPE program was seconded to ESARO for about 12 months in 1997 in order to help identify promising locations for piloting adaptations of the BRAC model.

UNICEF was by no means the only client for consulting services from NFPE staff. At the instigation of governments and national NGOs, senior NFPE staff participated in pro bono delegations to several countries, including Ethiopia, Pakistan, and India. As was the case for visitors to BRAC, neither BRAC nor its clients maintained systematic records of all their international consulting work. The following illustrative cases, therefore, are based largely on interviews with BRAC staff in 2007.

Oxfam America in South Asia. Among the people from dozens of countries coming to look at BRAC NFPE in the first half of the 1990s, one of the earliest was the regional representative for Oxfam America in South Asia. Following her visit to BRAC, the representative proposed that Oxfam support NFPE in many NGOs in India as soon as possible. Oxfam's board, however, limited Oxfam support to a pilot adaptation of the BRAC NFPE model by two local NGOs in two districts in India.

A study a few years later found that 1,800 children in 30 Oxfam-supported, BRAC-modeled nonformal centers were finishing Grade 3 and preparing to transfer into government schools (Varma & Malviya, 1996). Although the students in these centers were mainly dropouts or had never enrolled in school, the study reported that 90% of them—70% of them girls—had successfully completed primary education and continued their education in secondary schools.

Whether the success of this pilot project led to an expansion of community schools in India is not known. As was the case with almost all countries where BRAC provided short- or long-term consultants, BRAC subsequently lost contact with the two Indian NGOs that were adapting its NFPE model.[6]

UNICEF in Sierra Leone. During a workshop with regional UNICEF education staff in Senegal, a BRAC consultant was approached by a staff member from UNICEF's Sierra Leone office. The consultant recalled subsequently that the staff person was excited by the presentation and persuaded UNICEF to bring the consultant to Freetown to help launch an NFPE pilot. During the ensuing short-term consultancy, the BRAC consultant found that the UNICEF staffer had "thousands" of photocopies of one of the UNICEF-sponsored NFPE reports (Lovell & Fatema, 1989) stacked in her office. The staff person showed a keen appreciation of both the elements of BRAC's management model and the need to adapt them to Sierra Leone. The adaptation effort was under way when civil war started in Sierra Leone and BRAC's work with the NFPE effort in Sierra Leone was curtailed.

A BRAC consultant returned to Sierra Leone in 2001 or 2002, with a testing expert to help evaluate the state of the NFPE schools that had survived or been started after the war. Tests showed NFPE students doing better than the formal school students. The consultant commended the UNICEF officer for modifying the model to fit the Sierra Leone context, including hiring unemployed formal teachers to teach in their NFPE-type schools. In 2005 UNICEF reported that 400 of the community schools covering Grades 1 through 3 had served approximately 19,000 children and that by 2009, 900 more such schools would be established (Chiejine, 2005). As was the case in India, BRAC did not maintain contact with the Sierra Leone project.

Of her short-term consulting experience, Kaniz Fatema reflected, "In a short visit you cannot study things properly. I felt frustrated everywhere I went" (personal communication, Kaniz Fatema, December 12, 2006). Short-term consultancies did not permit sufficient time for BRAC staff to fully imagine the best ways the NFPE model might be adapted in other countries, particularly with respect to the complex management model. Moreover, without high-speed Internet and email access during the 1990s, and often with limited English as the only common language, following up short consultancies in writing was not practical. Long-term consultancies seemed to offer a better chance to help local organizations to adapt and establish new kinds of NFPE models and to stay with them long enough to get both school and management models on a solid footing.

Camping Out: Long-Term Consulting

In the late 1990s several UNICEF staff moved directly from water and sanitation projects in Bangladesh to staff UNICEF's Operation Lifeline [southern] Sudan (OLS). Because at that time southern Sudan lacked a formal government, UNICEF took an unusually active, hands-on role in OLS. The head of the OLS was unsatisfied with the "lack of new ideas" in southern Sudan and dispatched a group of about a dozen southern Sudanese on a study tour to Bangladesh, Nepal, and India. The UNICEF field program coordinator for education in OLS was impressed with the BRAC NFPE program and was determined to try it out in southern Sudan.

At the coordinator's request, BRAC sent a series of consultants to begin work in Rumbek. A small plane regularly flew international relief agency staff and materials from Kampala to a small town on the Uganda-Sudan border where most agencies maintained offices. From there a U.N. plane made the trip to Rumbek less frequently. Rumbek had few buildings or even building materials beyond handmade mud bricks; roofing material, furniture, and most supplies had to be flown in. BRAC consultants lived in tents, and water was rationed. In 2002, there was only one girl enrolled in the secondary school in Rumbek. In the widely dispersed, sparsely populated rural communities, most inhabitants with 8 or more years of education had left for the cities, draining the already small pool of paraprofessional teacher candidates.

In mid-2001, three short-term BRAC consultants participated in a 3-day strategic planning symposium organized by UNICEF and the southern Sudan provisional education authority. One of the BRAC consultants said that the presentation UNICEF asked them to prepare felt "like we were selling our program to them." The first longer-term BRAC consultant visited Rumbek in November 2001 and returned to begin a 6-month consultancy in March 2002. UNICEF invited potential staff to a seminar the consultant prepared on the BRAC model. From the seminar participants, the consultant selected two program officers, one materials developer, and one team leader. Together these staff set up 10 lower (Grades 1 through 3) primary schools during the first 6-month consultancy, with the consultant working alongside the staff to identify communities, students, teachers, and supplies, and to conduct training.

The Sudan environment demanded many adaptations of the BRAC classroom model:

- Educated women were hard to find in rural communities. Of the first 10 schoolteachers selected in southern Sudan, only 4 were women.

- All buildings were in full-time use. Consultants organized communities to make mud-brick shells and UNICEF flew in roofing material.
- No large mats of any material were available, so staff asked parents to send small mats for their children to sit on.
- Low population density meant that few communities had 30 eligible students within a 1-mile radius. Selecting only communities meeting this criterion meant a distance of 65 km between some schools. After trying this and finding it impractical, the minimum number of students was reduced and the catchment area was increased.
- Because of the distance between schools and the lack of roads, POs could not reach all schools weekly. POs responsible for very distant communities were issued camping equipment and arranged to spend several days at a time per month in harder-to-reach communities.

In addition, critical support services were lacking:

- Rumbek had no professional printers to produce learning materials. Staff photocopied and collated many materials by hand.
- UNICEF provided textbooks in the local language, Dinka, but teachers' guides and many learning materials that BRAC considered essential were not available. A short-term consultancy by a BRAC materials developer translated some materials from Bangla into English, but there was no one to translate them into Dinka.

In total, five consultants, including one woman, all of whom had 10 or more years of experience with BRAC, served for up to 6 months each over a 2-year period. Together with the newly hired southern Sudan authority staff, these consultants helped establish between 120 and 200 "Village Girls' Schools" in three areas. In addition, BRAC consultants also trained CARE and Save the Children staff in the BRAC NFPE model with the expectation that the three organizations together would be operating 600 schools by the end of 2004. Some or all of the CARE and Save the Children schools were later funded by USAID under the Sudan Basic Education Program.

The UNICEF/OLS education program officer returned to Bangladesh in 2003 to request a memorandum of understanding that would generate a steady stream of BRAC consultants into southern Sudan for several years. BRAC, however, now expanding into Afghanistan, lacked sufficient senior staff members to fulfill this request. When the UNICEF education program officer transferred out of southern Sudan in the middle of 2004 and was not replaced by someone similarly inspired to press the BRAC connection, BRAC staff lost touch with the program. Despite the advent of high-speed Internet and email access after 2000, up to 2007, written follow-up of the long-term, on-site coaching did not occur. This may have been at least in part a problem with limited English. As of 2008 some of the South Sudanese schools started by BRAC with UNICEF funding and supported by CARE and Save the Children with USAID funding were still in operation.

Reflecting on the various short-term advising and the Sudanese long-term coaching experiences, BRAC staff emphasized the importance of individual initiative within the requesting organization, Northern or Southern, governmental or nongovernmental. They concluded that someone had to have both vision and stamina to create and maintain the momentum necessary to launch the adaptation process and follow it through.

Moving In: Direct Implementation and Mentoring

At the beginning of the 21st century, BRAC was arguably the largest national nongovernmental organization in the world. In 2005, BRAC's revenue from commercial projects (such as the BRAC Bank) and program-support enterprises (such as handicrafts retailing) plus service charges for loans to village organization members totaled almost US$140 million,[7] more than twice the international donor grants it received that year (BRAC, 2006). This gave BRAC rare flexibility as a Southern NGO to pilot its own ideas and launch new programs without reference to Northern funders. This streamlined BRAC's work in microfinance, where interest payments could render a new program in a new country self-sustaining within a matter of years. There were no precedents for self-financing first-generation primary education, however, so government or donor funding had to be found.

Afghanistan. The 2001 fall of the Taliban in Afghanistan produced an outpouring of support for Afghan reconstruction from an unexpected source: Bangladesh. Excerpts from the memoir of a Bengali educator who worked in Kabul from 1927 to 1929 (Ali, 1948) had been required reading for several generations of secondary school and college students in Dhaka and kindled the imaginations of some. The geography of the two countries—one flat, densely populated, humid, and green, the other mountainous, sparsely populated, dry, and often brown—was vastly different. So were the cultures and languages. Yet BRAC staff compared the postwar status of Afghanistan in 2001 to the status of Bangladesh in 1971—infrastructure destroyed, refugees returning to devastated villages—and felt solidarity (Chowdhury, Alam, & Ahmed, 2006).

Shortly after the fall of the Taliban, therefore, Abed, now the chairman of BRAC, sent a group of senior managers on a fact-finding visit to Afghanistan. On a second visit later that year, Abed met with the Minister for Rural Reconstruction and Development (MRRD), who requested BRAC's help with a 5-year strategic plan. Still later that same year, BRAC began the process of registering as an international NGO; piloted programs in several sectors in two Afghan provinces (Parwan and Balkh); and conducted the surveys that helped determine BRAC's three priority sectors in Afghanistan: microfinance, health, and education. BRAC sent some of its most experienced managers to direct the Afghan work. It funded most of these start-ups with income from its profit-making enterprises in Bangladesh.

In 2002 BRAC launched 24 pilot schools for older girls in two Afghan provinces with funds from the Swedish International Development Cooperation Agency (SIDA). In addition, the UNICEF-funded Accelerated Learning (or Winter) Program provided BRAC with an opportunity to demonstrate the range of its capabilities in primary education to the Government of Afghanistan. Through the Accelerated Learning Program, BRAC helped nearly 15,000 older children to advance one grade in 4 months. This involved developing teacher training material; master trainers who would then train 159 Grade 2 teachers and 318 Grade 1 teachers during the winter months; and mathematics training for 500 teachers. In addition, BRAC established regular coordination with the Ministry of Education and UNICEF, and it trained and dispatched local supervisors to visit each school twice weekly (BRAC Education Programme, 2002).

In each of these endeavors, BRAC created a somewhat new school model, using different combinations of formal curricula and outside materials, and finding new ways to train female teachers in communities where few women were permitted to attend residential training. Bangladeshi staff reported that Afghan women were willing and able to do much more than their Afghan male colleagues were prepared at first to ask of them, much as had been the case in Bangladesh 20 years earlier. BRAC also had to adjust the pace of the curriculum for Afghan children who, having grown up in refugee camps and only recently returned to rural areas, had a broader exposure to the world and to print than most rural Bangladeshi children had.

Based on the track record established with the Accelerated Program, BRAC worked much more closely with the Ministry of Education in Afghanistan than it was able to with its counterpart in Bangladesh. Initially, the priority areas for primary education identified by the ministry—establishing formal primary school buildings and recruiting and paying professional teachers—appeared to clash with BRAC's commitment to minimal infrastructure, part-time paraprofessional teachers, and serving overage girls in rural areas. Later in 2004, UNICEF's former senior advisor to education, now working with BRAC, conducted a strategic planning meeting for teachers and government officials, during which a complementary role for BRAC within the formal government system began to emerge.

According to its annual report, by the end of 2005, BRAC had established 52 area offices in 26 districts in 13 provinces and had operated or was operating three types of schools: 608 2-year classes covering 3 years of the formal primary curriculum for older girls; 216 feeder schools providing 1 year of school readiness for young children; and 24 nonformal primary education schools. Under the Accelerated Learning Program, BRAC was continuing to provide basic teacher and extra mathematics training to 158 teachers. Under all these programs, 80% of the students and more than 80% of the teachers were female (BRAC, 2006). Because many of its schools existed for only 1 or 2 years, to help overage children catch up and rejoin formal primary schools, the exact number of schools BRAC continues to operate is difficult to estimate. As of April 2006, BRAC anticipated opening up to 5,000 new schools (Chowdhury, Alam, & Ahmed, 2006).

As of 2007, it seemed that building a primary education system in Afghanistan would require massive international assistance for a decade or more. In the context of international NGOs (INGOs) in Afghanistan, BRAC stood out as a low-cost partner with a good track record with key donors. As in southern Sudan, BRAC's Bangladeshi managers lived simply, in the Afghan rather than the expatriate community. In contrast with Western INGOs, BRAC spent little on security and paid Bangladeshi staff just twice their normal salary—a small fraction of a Western expatriate's salary supplemented by danger pay. The program had some tragic setbacks,[8] but continued to expand. Attacks on BRAC in the name of Islam by elites in Bangladesh more than a decade earlier informed the organization's response to religious extremism in Afghanistan. Over several years, as Afghans pick up experience, confidence, and something of the BRAC organizational culture, senior BRAC staff said, they plan to increase the number of Afghan managers and reduce the number of Bangladeshi staff in Afghanistan.

Uganda. BRAC also launched a country office in Uganda in 2006 and that same year responded to requests from the government for education for children in internally displaced persons camps. One of NFPE's most experienced senior staff moved to Uganda to head the BRAC office and oversaw the development of 122 "second chance" schools for children 10 to 15 years old and older adolescent girls who had become child mothers. The program offered accelerated learning to help older children catch up quickly and rejoin mainstream schools. When the camps closed in 2008 and 2009, BRAC moved with camp residents into villages and started 265 schools, offering instruction for younger children as well. By 2010, BRAC was the largest nongovernment organization in Uganda, disbursing US$24 million in microfinance in 2009 for more than 150,000 members of microfinance groups.

In summary, the size of BRAC's independent operating budget and the size of its staff in Bangladesh gave it the luxury of diverting staff and resources to a new country, to set up operations first and find donor funding later. In connection with tsunami relief, it also set up a small international office in Sri Lanka; its work there included some support to local schools. Other offices in Tanzania and, subsequently, South Sudan managed an East African health initiative for the Gates Foundation and operated schools for children and accelerated learning, livelihood training, and health outreach for adolescent girls. In contrast with Afghanistan, however, few donors in these places were looking for partners to scale-up basic education for children or adolescents. Yet BRAC was invited to open an office in Pakistan, where more international support for education was likely to be forthcoming. The establishing of BRAC offices in Asia and Africa helped national staff in those countries experience not just the BRAC NFPE school model, but also its management model and the trial-and-error approach to program design. Self-financing meant that BRAC could afford to keep experienced Bangladeshi managers in these countries until such time as nationals were deemed ready to take over operations, even if it should take, as BRAC staff suggested in southern Sudan, a decade or more.

CONCLUSIONS

As with scaling up in one context, scaling out into other new contexts may have been easier for the health innovation ORT than for the education innovation NFPE. But by no means was it simple. "Seeing is believing" mobilized early adopters and witnesses in Dhaka and Calcutta to carry the ORS gospel to other countries. Committed high-status scientists were faster carriers of innovation than international peer-reviewed publications, but the latter provided strong legitimation. Widespread adoption of ORT in new countries demanded major investments in market research and qualitative studies to tailor ORT to local conditions and organizations. Getting an immunization is a largely passive, one-time affair; in contrast, ORT demands learning, behavior change, decisionmaking, and, at times, sustained action under pressure—persuading a child or adult to keep sipping ORS even though the patient may continue to vomit and experience diarrhea for hours more. Both quantitative and qualitative research were marshaled to identify local words for different types of diarrhea; the sorts of containers available in the home for mixing ORS; cultural beliefs and norms about diarrhea; packet color and graphics preferences; and more. Randomized controlled trials, the most highly legitimated test of social interventions, played a modest, supporting role. Still, humanitarian crises continued to be the first places where ORT came into wide use. Even in those circumstances, the treatment sometimes met resistance, as was the case in the disaster relief operation in Goma.

Scaling out both ORS and NFPE in new countries followed a pattern similar to the one discussed in Chapters 4 and 5: *imagining* how something from one context might be used in another; *adapting* it in that context for effectiveness and cost-effectiveness; and *further adapting* it, at least throughout much of the beginning of a new scaling up phase. The main difference encountered in scaling out was that, unlike Bangladesh, few countries constitute a single context; that is, most countries comprise multiple ethnic groups, some speaking mutually unintelligible languages, and inhabiting distinct ecological environments. This calls for some—often major—adaptation of the core deliverable to complement the available delivery agents and delivery systems. Scaling up nationally may require more than one organization in order to reach all the contexts in a single country. In addition, scaling up in some smaller contexts—as BRAC discovered in its more recent efforts to serve the hard-to-reach ethnic and linguistic minorities in Bangladesh—may require more extensive adaptation and be much more costly. It may be necessary, for example, to translate, test, and print Grade 1 and part of Grade 2 textbooks in a second language, add a teacher's helper who speaks the mother tongue to each Grade 1 classroom, and so on. Reaching 90% of the population with a single low-cost deliverable and delivery system is not likely to be replicated in much of Africa.

The bottleneck to expansion and to quality improvement in some contexts, as in Bangladesh, was the availability and quality of delivery agents. In Bangladesh ineffective or unreliable POs and teachers were promptly replaced; in many other, less densely populated places with lower levels of education, such as southern Sudan, this was not practical. For ORT, expatriate scientists were paid at international rates, allowing them to live relatively comfortably, with their families, in expatriate communities in major cities. For NFPE, there was a limited pool of capable middle or senior managers with the necessary implicit knowledge who were willing to be stationed overseas in difficult countries for 6 months at a time without their families. In a backhanded way, recent interest in "implementation science" in public health demonstrates the degree to which scaling up public health programs continues to rely on implicit knowledge embodied in experienced middle and senior managers. This suggest the first generalization relating to scaling out in new contexts:

C6.1. Managers/experts who have hands-on experience scaling up an innovation in one context are willing to take up residence and assist with the adaptation and scaling up of that innovation in another context.

The process of scaling out into new countries described in this chapter was largely consistent with the working hypotheses laid out in the previous chapter. ORS and NFPE scaled out further in countries where some organization(s) already delivered some services to the target areas, whether it be a government ministry or an NGO. To some extent, Oxfam in India and Save the Children in Malawi and Mali made NFPE possible on a small and large scale, respectively. In southern Sudan, absent an implementing organization, no amount of enthusiasm or funding on the part of UNICEF staff could call forth a school system. In the same context, CARE International and Save the Children, with funding from USAID and some training from NFPE, managed to keep some community schools going in southern Sudan after the departure of BRAC, but no organization was in place to scale-up further when USAID funding ended.

The discussion above, however, suggests that the factors that help increase the speed of scaling out into a new context are not so different from those for scaling up in one context, save one:

C6.2. The target context or a significant number of delivery sites are relatively free from external conflict.

At least two factors have made it difficult for other countries to capitalize on BRAC's innovation in NFPE. First, the power of the Western model of mass primary schooling remains paramount. This model tends to devalue other ways of organizing education, except in emergencies where other models may be tolerated as stopgap or catching-up strategies, as BRAC demonstrated in Ugandan refugee camps and among recently former refugees returning to rural Afghanistan. However, by 2004, the Interagency[9] Network for Emergency Education (f. 2000, INEE) released standards for emergency education, clearly trying to bring even stopgap schools into line with the world model (Bromley & Andina, 2009). This chapter reinforces the notion that any school or school system that does not hew closely to the Western model—professional teacher, age-graded classrooms, constructivist pedagogy, learning resource–rich classrooms—operates at a distinct disadvantage and will have difficulty scaling up or out.

Second, where BRAC's NFPE works, it is largely because it is a complete system. In Chapter 4, a senior manager said he liked Kaniz's model because BRAC was in control of every aspect (personal communication, M.

Aminul Alam, January 28, 2007). But most organizations are not willing or able to implement all aspects of the program. Although most visitors see a single classroom in a building that looks like all the rest in the village, with a teacher with a secondary school education and a simplified curriculum, this is the tip of the iceberg of the NFPE program. That classroom and teacher are backed up by weekly visits by a college-educated young man or woman on a bicycle or motorcycle who delivers textbooks and teaching and learning materials, follows up on absences, and keeps parents engaged. And that young man or woman is backed up with a support system that provides him with that motorcycle and a place to live and a supervisor, and three layers of monitoring and auditing and textbooks and training and interface with donors and the public and people to raise funds from foreigners. The school model, therefore, may be simple, but the system that backs it up is complete and, as such, complex. Where BRAC has been able to establish a country office, complete with long-term staff and delivery support services, it has generally been able to adapt one of its school models to the local context and, within a year or two, offer an education that is of good quality by local standards. As for developing local staff into diligent POs and somewhat autonomous middle managers? Even BRAC itself needs more time for that.

Given the relative rarity of local organizations with the sort of comprehensive mix of competencies BRAC has developed, why don't First World educators and international development organizations promote some innovation simpler than a full primary education? Remembering the importance of different discourse in different periods, such an approach, clearly, might run afoul of a strict interpretation of the "country-ownership" development norm noted at the beginning of this chapter. Moreover, it would demand a critical mass in the EFA community reconciling itself to a more selective approach to an already selective goal, not just to primary education but to some necessary but not sufficient component of a full primary education. The next chapter provides a case study of the emergence of such an innovation, or at least an "innovative" indicator, in the decade or so leading up to 2015.

CHAPTER 7

Reimagining
What Can Data Do?

Throughout the cases laid out in the previous chapters, data—that is, evidence that can be summarized in quantitative form—have played an important role both in defining crises and in attempting to mobilize large-scale international action around them. In Chapter 2, professionals in international organizations used cross-national data to convince many in the industrialized and less industrialized world that the deaths of so many children before age 5 was morally unacceptable when cheap and effective innovations to prevent those deaths were close at hand. In Chapter 3, the abrupt drop in mortality rates for cholera persuaded many in the scientific and the lay communities to adopt Oral Rehydration Therapy. In Chapter 4, BRAC used results from the chloride concentration test to prove to many skeptics that a homemade version of ORS was safe and effective. In Chapter 5, BRAC attempted to use enrollment, attendance, and transition rates to demonstrate the effectiveness of its alternative school model, as well as the effectiveness of the Assessment of Basic Competencies and the *Education Watch* assessment. In Chapter 6, national oral rehydration programs conducted surveys to buttress every aspect of their work. Up to this point, I have argued that in comparison with the education sector, the health sector has generated better data and used them more effectively in building support for innovations that, in turn, gained traction for a global goal.

This chapter describes the efforts of international development professionals to institutionalize a more compelling indicator of education quality: Early Grades Reading Assessments (EGRA). As described below, EGRA aimed to help the sector design and identify quicker, better, and cheaper primary education interventions, which, in turn, would gain more traction for better-quality primary education for all. The approach is selective because in the context of UPE, the early grades constitute just two or three of the five or six grades in conventional primary school. Likewise, reading, although necessary for all other school learning, is just one of six or seven required subjects in most primary curricula. Nonetheless, EGRA introduces new data into the discussion of when and how to use unconventional innovations in support of EFA. In some ways, EGRA resembles the first of four activities constituting the Child Survival initiative: growth monitoring. Neither is an end in itself: both are designed to measure performance against norms; and neither, alone, can correct the shortfalls they reveal. However, both have the capacity to move the discussion in their respective sector onto more technical ground, where professionals who exercise more jurisdiction, with the right evidence, can sometimes shake loose hundreds of millions of dollars in new funding.

Child Survival continues to serve as an effective mobilizing tool for a selective version of HFA (Bryce, Victora, & Black, 2013). Could early reading provide a similarly promising if selective approach to make faster progress toward the primary education component of EFA? Table 7.1 represents such a thought experiment, imagining early reading analogs to each component of GOBI: after-school remedial classes; early childhood education; extra time for reading in the curriculum and time on task in the classroom; and community libraries, to name a few. Consistent with earlier cases, there are, of course, no universal models for any of these reading interventions, but several NGOs have already moved beyond low-cost field experiments and into large-scale pilots for each of these activities in a half-dozen countries.

Table 7.1. The Selective Approach: Comparing Child Survival Initiative with Early Grades Reading

Comprehensive Approach	Health for All	Education for All
Selective version	Child Survival and Development Revolution	Universal Primary Education
Selective indicator	Children Under-5 Mortality Rate	Universal Primary Education Completion
Quality measure	Growth monitoring	Early grade reading & math assessments
Treatment	Oral rehydration therapy	After-school remedial reading & mathematics classes
Maintenance	Breastfeeding	Daily in-class time for reading & mathematics instruction
Prevention	Immunization	Early childhood education
Supplementation	Food supplementation: Vitamin A, iodine, zinc	After-school reading programs, community libraries
Changing attitudes	Female education	Female education
Reducing overall demands on the system	Family planning	Delay marriage/childbearing through female secondary education

Like all innovations described in this book, the adaptation and scaling up of an innovative indicator for primary education quality demanded a significant amount of agency and action on the part of individuals, whether to construct and defend or to critique and resist. For simplicity's sake, only three individuals are highlighted in this narrative, but many others played important roles. Some of the most effective tools at the disposal of these individuals were preexisting models, blueprints, identities, and scripts, including cross-national comparisons of development indicators, time-limited development projects, international panels of education experts to establish global standards, and international development professionals as champions to mobilize the international development field and to move politicians.

HALFWAY TO 2010: "THEY CAN'T READ . . ."

At the same time the international community was already in the process of agreeing on an MDG for education measured in terms of years of school completed, a paper by a World Bank economist, "Where Has All the Education Gone?" (Pritchett, 2001), began to undermine the tidy notion that years of schooling was a reasonable proxy for learning. That paper was followed by a series of retrospective reviews of the primary education portfolios of some of the most active donors to primary education. For the most part these reviews concluded that in terms of student learning, the "impact" of donor "investments" was either impossible to measure or negligible (Al-Samarrai, Bennell, & Colclough, 2002, U.K. Department for International Development [DfID]; Chapman, 2001, UNICEF; Chapman & Quijada, 2008, USAID; World Bank, Independent Evaluation Group, 2006). The author of the most recent of these reports described the difficulties of drawing conclusions from 33 independent evaluations, covering US$733 million spent between 1995 and 2005, of which

> 28 identified raising educational quality as a stated goal. Of those, 17 proposed student learning as a key indicator of educational quality. Of these, available data suggest that 12 actually measured student learning, of which 11 used pre- and post-testing to assess change over time. Of these 11, 9 designed the testing in a way that would support claims that student learning changes over time as a result of the project intervention (e.g., used a comparison group). Of these, 5 projects found meaningful increases in learning as a result of the project intervention. Another 3 found mixed results. . . . In 1 additional case the results were not clearly enough reported to interpret. (Chapman & Quijada, 2008, p. 5)

After 2005, well-circulated studies published by the World Bank and the [U.S.] National Bureau for Economic Research concluded that learning has a much stronger influence on national development than completed years of schooling (Hanushek & Woessmann, 2007, 2009). These conclusions, along with the primary education portfolio reviews, claimed to demonstrate that 15 years of funding for EFA had much less impact on economic growth than previously assumed. The findings, along with the lackluster EFA progress report in 2000 (UNESCO, 2000a, 2000b), led some observers, the present author included, to wonder whether the modest achievements of EFA and the findings of these retrospectives would end education's brief run as a leading actor on the global development stage.

Several professionals inside the World Bank and elsewhere, however, were already exploring a new approach to measure and address learning more directly. A psychologist in the Independent Evaluation Group[1] of the World Bank, Helen Abadzi, secured a grant from the Swiss government to study why so many adult literacy classes—a perennial component of most community development efforts—were producing so few literate adults. She enlisted the help of a psychologist at the University of Massachusetts at Amherst who suggested a link between this finding and a limitation of the brain: working memory absorbs seven items in about 12 seconds. The implication for adult literacy classes was that students needed to read one word every 1 to 1.5 seconds with 95% accuracy in order to understand the meaning of a sentence. Few adult literacy classes, however, provided either enough time on task for adults to reach that level of fluency or enough practice to achieve that degree of accuracy (Abadzi, 2008; Royer, Abadzi, & Kinda, 2004).

Abadzi saw the possible connection between the working memory issue and the low levels of achievement she was observing in her work on the World Bank's primary education portfolio review. She began compiling a report—soon a book—that would introduce professionals working in education and development to relatively new research in cognitive science and its implications for learning (Bransford, Brown, & Pellegrino, 2000). During an evaluation in Niger in 2004, she emailed her education colleagues in the World Bank,

> The Bank has leveraged much of Niger's education budget for the past 20 years. . . . In classes outside Niamey *none of the sampled students were found to be functionally literate.* . . . Teachers typically estimated that 30–50% knew how to read. But even the 6th graders graduating in three weeks read haltingly and did not know enough French to understand the texts or answer content questions. (email communication, Helen Abadzi to EDUFAM, June 29, 2004)

She suggested that World Bank education staff begin measuring learning and conduct rapid but systematic classroom level surveys to build a more actionable picture of what was happening in the lower grades of primary schools. To measure learning, she proposed oral reading fluency tests. These, she argued, were a) quick and cheap, and b) correlated closely with later reading comprehension.

Rapid oral reading fluency tests had enormous advantages for those trying to improve learning in countries with the farthest to go to meet EFA goals. Compared with paper-and-pencil national exams or cross-national achievement tests, such as the PISA and PIRLS assessments in which an increasing number of upper- and middle-income countries participate, oral reading and mathematics tests have many advantages, if for a narrower range of skills. Oral tests require much less assessment infrastructure and can be developed and administered much more quickly and, with proper training, with high levels of reliability. The cross-national examinations take years to plan, launch, analyze, and publish; oral tests, depending on their size, can be developed, administered to a nationally representative sample, and published in months. Paper-and-pencil tests are not valid for children who cannot yet read with comprehension and so are often not administered until Grade 3 or 4, by which time many children who are not learning have dropped out; oral tests can be given as early as preschool. In Bangladesh, where stipends are used to motivate students to enroll and remain in primary schools, on average about 20% of students who enroll in Grade 1 drop out before Grade 5. Combined with enrollment rates of around 90%, at least 30% of Bangladeshi children of primary school age do not complete primary school (World Bank, Human Development Sector, South Asia Region, 2013). Advocates argue that oral reading fluency tests can identify student progress and difficulties in Grades 1 and 2, raising the possibility of remediation before struggling students fall so far behind that dropout becomes inevitable.[2] For many ministries of education and international development professionals who were struggling with low levels of achievement and high levels of dropout, this was a compelling theory of change.

Luis Crouch, an economist then with the Research Triangle Institute International (f. 1956, RTI) in North Carolina,[3] read the draft of Abadzi's growing manuscript and suggested "60 words per minute" was a catchier phrase than one word per second. Abadzi began recording children reading for 1 minute at a time and played back these oral reading fluency tests to policy makers to demonstrate what she considered the dire state of learning in many primary schools. Working in Peru in 2004 and 2005, Crouch presented a slightly changed passage from the official Grade 1 language textbook, asked children to read a brief passage, and then asked them to answer three comprehension questions. Only 25% of Grade 1 students and 54% of

Grade 2 students could read one or more words. Those who read averaged only 9 or 29 correct words per minute, respectively. At that reading speed, comprehension tended to be compromised, and reading so slowly is, in any case, inefficient. The authors concluded,

> Worldwide, actions can be taken so that all children (particularly in countries with phonetically spelled languages[4]) can read fluently by the end of Grade 2. A rapid reading test administered quickly and inexpensively produced comprehensible and actionable information on student performance. If sampling and instrumentation were refined, the methodology could produce baseline and monitoring data that are locally sustainable and internationally comparable. (Abadzi et al., 2005, p. 137)

In Peru and soon in Nicaragua, the private sector became intrigued with the measure, and the World Bank and DfID funded a short video emphasizing the importance of children learning to read and comprehend at least 60 words per minute by the end of Grade 2. The video was created to use as a public announcement on national TV,[5] but staff in the Ministry of Education and leaders in the education community rejected both the message and the pedagogical approach it implied: spending more time on foundation skills,[6] including phonics and practice, to increase automaticity. However, the more basic recommendation, that reading should be measured early (Grade 2), at a time when remediation is still easy, was adopted by the government. At the same time, teachers' unions were convinced that any quantitative measure of learning could be used against them, so the ministry did not set a goal in terms of specific number of words correctly read per minute.

This work was being carried out at the same time and in the same department as the World Bank's primary education portfolio review (World Bank, Independent Evaluation Group, 2006). At the beginning of the 21st century, most educators would have preferred a more flexible, nuanced method for measuring learning achievement in EFA. However, improving oral reading fluency through greater emphasis on foundational skills appeared to be one of the few approaches to improving learning that was both doable and rapidly effective.

FROM ORAL READING FLUENCY TO EARLY GRADES READING

Abadzi presented some of her findings at the Comparative and International Education Society meetings in Salt Lake City in 2004, widening the discussion of early reading to include education professionals and scholars beyond the World Bank. In 2005, she attended an international literacy conference at Cambridge University and there met psychologists using 1-minute tests to measure reading fluency. She also began to tap into scholarly articles and concepts in cognitive science, such as psycholinguistic grain size[7] (Ziegler & Goswami, 2005), and began incorporating them into her book (Abadzi, 2006) in an effort to raise the level of discussion around early reading among international development professionals onto a more scientific plane.

Meanwhile, Crouch continued to look for projects and organizations that might expand the early reading work. The first opportunity came at the beginning of 2006 with a request from the Bill and Melinda Gates Foundation (f. 1997, the Gates Foundation) for a concept note for an international initiative in education. Up to that time, its international work focused on public health, but, like many international public health organizations, the foundation argued that education, particularly girls' education, multiplied the effect of maternal and child health interventions. Crouch was not an education specialist, so he recruited Amber Gove, an education economist with whom he had worked on the World Bank's primary education portfolio review. The concept note that they crafted identified three potential strategic areas for support, the first and most passionate being early reading skills. They wrote:

> Acquisition of basic reading in the early grades is the education equivalent of childhood immunizations: just as vaccines guarantee against future illness, learning to read fluently in the early grades is a minimum requirement for future success . . . . *There are simple, known, and inexpensive methods for teaching children to read,* yet they are not being systematized, distributed, and implemented in either teacher training institutions or schools. (Crouch & Gove, 2006, p. 2, emphasis added)

There were indeed simple, known, and inexpensive methods for teaching children to read. However, many countries lacked educationists who were familiar with the 1990s learning research and were able to adapt those methods and to integrate them into national curricula and teaching and learning materials, not to mention the matter of ministries or NGOs capable of piloting and scaling up relevant innovations. At a minimum, this suggested that each country would have to seek out existing approaches to foster automaticity and adapt them to as many languages and contexts as existed in each country.

With respect to early reading, Crouch and Gove's concept paper identified NGOs as the main source of innovation.

> Many of these programs have decades of experience and thousands of graduates; some programs also have demonstrated evidence of gains—in a few cases

the evidence is fairly rigorous. But these gains have never been *systematically* evaluated, and *generally* the evaluations are not rigorous enough. Furthermore, the pedagogical techniques they use are not sufficiently widespread, so the international community cannot see a clear package of practices that are known to work. (Crouch & Gove, 2006, author emphasis, p. 2)

Crouch and Gove acknowledged here that the existing technology did not yet meet the most rigorous scientific standards, but they assumed there were preexisting practices that were at least partway there. They also assumed, at least in the case of education, that a package of practices, not a stand-alone, one-time intervention, was most likely to be involved.

Their strategy proposed building consensus among the main organizations and professionals already active in the field in five steps:

1. Convene a meeting of experts, practitioners, and NGOs to identify the size and nature of the problem and agree upon potential solutions.
2. Invite experts and practitioners to identify promising strategies for teaching children to read based on a combination of existing research evidence and the practical experience of NGOs.
3. Fund selected designs as demonstration projects in several countries and contexts.
4. Standardize research designs across all projects (randomized selection, baseline measurement, and value-added scores in both treatment and control groups, where possible) to monitor progress throughout implementation.
5. Disseminate the findings so as to strongly erode the mentality that "it can't be done."

The Gates Foundation eventually issued a one-time request for proposals, mirroring the concept note, "to identify, implement and document scalable and cost-effective approaches to improve the quality of learning outcomes in the developing world." The request said that the foundation planned one-time grants for 5 to 10 proposals totaling at least $40 million, the goal being "to demonstrate, validate and establish strategies that can be dramatically increased in scale—both within a country and across country borders" within 3 to 5 years (Bill and Melinda Gates Foundation, 2006). The approach allowed enough time for adapting and small scale expansion in one context, but probably not for the sort of inventing, scaling up across a complete context, or scaling out to other contexts described in earlier chapters. RTI proposed partnering with largely national NGOs already engaged in piloting early reading interventions in six countries.

Although the Gates Foundation addressed its request to a small number of organizations, the request soon reached many more, and the foundation's small international education group was quickly overwhelmed with proposals. Later in 2006, the Gates Foundation handed most of its education funds over to the William and Flora Hewlett Foundation (f. 1971, Hewlett Foundation) to administer and select implementing partners. The Hewlett Foundation, in turn, also followed a strategy—Quality Education in Developing Countries (f. 2006, QEDC)—that incorporated most of the same elements as RTI's five-point proposal. The Hewlett Foundation had already supported the first of the five points through funding two earlier projects.[8] Hewlett therefore focused the Gates funding on Points 2 through 5 of the concept note, starting with awarding most of the funds to NGOs based in the global South, including two of RTI's proposed partners, in three of the six countries proposed by RTI. No funding went to RTI. Later the Hewlett Foundation awarded grants to international organizations, including RTI, to design and implement "rigorous" evaluations, including randomized controlled trials for the most systematic of the innovations. Each grantee partnered with a different evaluating organization and adopted a different research design. Ultimately, generalizations could not be drawn from these studies (McEwan, 2013).

RTI continued to implement many of the measurement ideas from the Gates proposal under an existing contract with USAID, EDDATA.[9] The source of these funds had important implications for the activities that came to be associated with early grades reading (EGR) (Chabbott, 2006). EDDATA funds could only be used for measuring EGR or comparing innovations at the pilot stage, not for medium- or large-scale reading interventions. The funds offered cost-sharing and technical assistance to USAID missions in Nicaragua, Jamaica, Peru, and South Africa. In 2007 the World Bank began funding similar work for ministries of education in Senegal and the Gambia. In keeping with concerns about "country-led" development and government "autonomy," the World Bank aimed to help develop effective administrative systems that would hold service providers accountable to governments. The bank had no clear position on how people learn, particularly marginalized students, so it funded inputs, such as textbooks, and emphasized school autonomy and testing. Governments and school officials were expected to discover on their own how to teach students most effectively (Helen Abadzi, personal communication, May 14, 2014).

In November 2006, with support from the World Bank and USAID, RTI convened the first of several biennial meetings, as it earlier had proposed to Gates. Thirteen reading researchers and practitioners from four countries with 14 observers from international development organizations gathered in a small conference room at the World Bank to propose approaches to

measuring standards for testing reading in the early grades. RTI was specifically looking for advice on the design of two types of EGRA: one simple and
another more comprehensive. The experts found the work to date funded
by donors and other work initiated by NGOs interesting and appropriate. They recommended that both the simple and the more comprehensive
EGRA include several subtests. The notion of a universal measure based on
words per minute was neither rejected nor recommended. They referred to
well-known tools such as the DIBELS (Dynamic Indicators of Basic Early
Learning Skills), CTOPP (Comprehensive Test of Phonological Processing),
and the Woodcock-Johnson Tests of Achievement, among others. They also
considered some lesser-known tools, such as an assessment of reading fluency based on assessor judgment rather than time, developed by the Indian
NGO Pratham. Following the meeting, RTI began using the term EGRA[10]
for any combination of rapid foundation reading skills subtests administered from preschool through Grade 4. Although often associated with RTI,
the term EGRA is not copyrighted.

Prior to this time, RTI had used EGRA mainly on a small scale for
"reading snapshots" and as an instrument for classroom-based assessments.
In 2007, building on the workshop recommendations, RTI began to use
EGRA for at least two other purposes: as a rigorous national or system-
level diagnostic and as an impact evaluation tool for a single program or
project (Gove & Wetterberg, 2011). Abadzi took another tack, using systematic classroom observation to find out how classroom time was spent
(Abadzi, 2007). These findings helped tease out which existing teaching approaches resulted in the biggest gains in reading fluency in underresourced
classrooms; explored what types of community participation were feasible
in largely illiterate communities; identified and analyzed potential gains
from remedial reading programs (Schwartz, 2011); and identified quicker,
less expensive ways of producing quality textbooks and other teaching and
learning materials relevant to reading.

EGRA was intended to be used as a template, not a blueprint. Ideally,
for each context, only a subset of a dozen or so potential subtests would
be selected, adapted, and developed in—not replicated or translated into—
local languages. RTI and other organizations willing to take an open-source
approach used the EDDATA website to disseminate free, downloadable versions of EGRA in many languages, from any organization willing to share
them. In principle, this was useful and easy to understand, but in practice,
though much less complex than for cross-national large-scale assessments,
such as the pre-Progress in International Reading Literacy Study assessment,[11] test implementation was complex. In most cases, additional unique
local content, instructions, and training materials for test administrators
had to be created on-site for each language and context. However, few of

those responsible for developing these assessments—ministry, donor, and NGO professionals—had any background in cognitive psychology, statistics, and linguistics. In addition, few could handle the complex development and implementation of seven or eight early reading subtests. Finally, insistence on rigor and on "all"—implying more subgroup analysis and larger samples—clashed with the need to keep the assessments quick and simple. RTI, therefore, was contracted to design and implement EGRA in many countries. Similarly, at the request of donors, RTI also created teams, including domestic and international reading experts, statisticians, and policy dialogue specialists, to conduct workshops at the country and regional level as well as in Washington for donor organization staff to introduce them to better assessment methods.

Demand grew quickly for step-by-step instructions for preparing local professionals to conduct valid program or national-level EGRA. By 2007 Gove had drafted and was circulating a pilot version of a step-by-step, 88-page *EGRA Toolkit* (Gove, 2009) in English; later it was released in Spanish and French versions. The purpose of the toolkit was narrow: to develop a sample-based "system diagnostic" to inform ministries and donors. Using EGRA for high-stakes decisions, whether for funding or for individual students, was strongly discouraged (p. 6). The demand for specific instructions remained high, and a 98-page *Guidance Notes for Planning and Implementing EGRA* followed 5 years later (Research Triangle Institute & International Rescue Committee, 2012) on the EDDATA site. By the end of 2010, many organizations had designed and implemented various types and versions of EGRA, in more than 70 languages in over 40 countries, about half of them funded by USAID and the rest with other donor, national government, or NGO support (Gove & Cvelich, 2010). Many of these assessments were quite different from or predated the battery of tests included in Gove's toolkit, but they had not captured the attention of policymakers previously. In some cases, different versions of EGRA conducted in the same country helped to validate each other.

IMAGINING THE PARALLELS WITH HEALTH

The G in GOBI stands for growth monitoring, a process that *measures* children's height, weight, and upper arm circumference periodically, from birth to age 5 or 6. The purpose of the measurement is to identify children who are undernourished or suffering chronic disease *so that* their caregivers can address those issues before the children's health is permanently compromised. Similarly, at the classroom level, EGRA *measures* young children's reading progress and identifies those who are not making timely progress, ideally *so that* teachers can provide appropriate remediation before children fall so far behind that they are unable to catch up.

Both growth monitoring and EGRA utilize simple, widely available instruments: scales, tape measures, growth charts in the case of the former and stopwatches and test booklets for each student in the latter. Both measures compare results to previously established "normal" ranges, by age in the former case or portion of the school year and language in the latter.[12] Both measures are leading indicators but not *the* leading indicator or a comprehensive measure of either robust child health or a quality primary education. Both measures must be adapted to each context and language. Growth monitoring charts, for example, must take into account genetic and environmental variation by context; the ideal growth trajectory varies a great deal between the diminutive Bushmen/San of Southern Africa and the tall but slim Masai in East Africa. These growth trajectories are, of course, works in progress as diet and living conditions change over time.

Both growth monitoring and EGRA also have a linguistic element. The correct words for critical conditions relative to children's physical well-being and disease, such as commonly used words for different types of diarrhea, must be identified or invented for each context. Similarly, EGRA instruments, training materials, and field manuals must be thoroughly adapted for each language and context, ideally maintaining some comparability across both. Finally, in most contexts, low levels of income are consistently associated with bigger gaps between national benchmarks and children's actual patterns of physical and cognitive growth.

Neither growth monitoring nor EGRA has a direct effect on children's growth or reading achievement. In fact, the earliest and loudest demands for data from these two measures were from development program managers, who needed authoritative indicators to report on program progress to donor organizations. Demand for indicators from busy teachers and illiterate parents, who, with the right training, could conceivably use them to improve reading instruction or provide more time on task for reading, were much less urgent. However, under the organizational pressures described in earlier chapters, both measures were all too easily transformed into sticks by which to hold field staff, or projects, or organizations accountable to overly optimistic quantitative goals set at the global, national plan, and project levels. Such pressures tend to "weaponize" any quantitative performance indicator used to establish targets at the beginning of a program, hence the resistance of the Peruvian teachers' union to "60 words per minute." As described in Chapters 4 through 6, from kitchen-sink experiments to scaling out to other countries, all innovations advance with a certain amount of trial, error, and failure and therefore require multiple indicators and flexibility in targets.

Both growth monitoring and EGRA became more like interventions where they were used for social mobilization. For child survival, this involved encouraging caretakers to note when the child was not growing within the average range and to take action within the scope of their existing resources. For example, mothers might administer ORS and food at the first sign of diarrhea; breast-feed longer and start appropriate solid foods sooner; and bring all children, both boys and girls, for vaccinations and booster shots at the right age.

Similarly, some education measurement efforts, like Read India and the related Uwezo in Kenya, publicized poor results from rapid oral assessments of early reading and mathematics, along with a short list of actions parents and local school authorities could take to improve learning. The messages for parents included: encourage your child to read aloud to you at home; send your child to school every day, on time; administer a simple reading test to your child; attend parent-teacher meetings. Monthly visits to a clinic for growth monitoring or to the school for parents' meetings constituted ideal times to promote and follow up on these actions. However, few ministries of health or education in the lowest-income countries had the capacity to support field agents to carry out these visits and follow up. For both Child Survival and EGR, social marketing—through radio, posters, traveling theater, and music ensembles—was not as effective as face-to-face social mobilization, but in many cases it was the only feasible strategy.

The global goal of child survival remained more compelling than that of survival to Grade 5 or 6 in primary school, or its completion. Nonetheless, similar criticisms have been leveled at both: simply surviving to age 5 or Grade 5 does not guarantee an acceptable quality of a child's life or cognition. Child Survival and early grade reading proponents respond that the only way to ensure the quality of life or education is to measure early and often and make available interventions to address deficits as they are observed. Growth monitoring and EGRA are, therefore, necessary but not sufficient indicators for a quality life or quality education.

As we saw in earlier chapters, innovations to improve child survival were developed in use-oriented laboratories and by NGOs working in the global South. There were no such laboratories for primary education. By 2005, however, some NGOs had started developing innovations in education interventions in the contexts that had farthest to go to achieve EFA goals. Unfortunately, potential funders for those innovations, specifically large philanthropies such as the Hewlett Foundation, were reluctant to make the long-term investments in use-oriented research or in the lengthy trial-and-error approach typically used by NGOs in the adaptation and scaling up processes. Instead, several funders, driven by the fast-approaching

2015 deadline for the MDGs, focused on RCTs in the hope of finding proven innovations that could scale-up quickly.

NON-GOVERNMENT ORGANIZATIONS (NGOs): THE LINK BETWEEN EARLY GRADES READING ASSESSMENTS AND READING IMPROVEMENT

Improved EGR instruction in primary school has been a component of many national and international development projects for decades under a variety of projects, as have oral reading fluency tests.[13] Each of the NGO interventions described below contained some elements but not all of the following commitments that characterized later efforts to improve reading instruction:

- *The 5 Ts: teachers* trained to teach reading; sufficient *textbooks* and leveled reading material; *time* on task for reading; attention to mother *tongue*; and frequent, low-stakes *testing* (Gove & Cvelich, 2010).
- *Prompt action*: for children who are not performing on the same level as their peers, remediation or enrichment either during or after school hours.
- *Social mobilization*: involving communities in supporting children's literacy in school and in the community (Gove & Cvelich, 2010).
- *Rigorous research*: to establish the cost-effectiveness of interventions.

How Molteno Intervened

An early study by the Molteno Institute for Language and Literacy (f. 1974, South Africa, Molteno)[14] concluded that many children in South African primary schools were failing to learn to read in English largely because they did not speak it and because English has one of the most complex, irregular spelling systems of any language. As of early 2013, Molteno had developed EGR intervention in the form of learning materials, and had provided training and mentorship to newly recruited teachers for mother-tongue and English-development programs throughout South Africa and eight other African countries.

By the first decade of the 21st century, most early literacy specialists agreed that children who did not speak the language of instruction when they entered Grade 1 should learn to read in their mother tongue while simultaneously learning to speak and build vocabulary in the language of instruction (Abadzi, 2006; Brock-Utne, 2007; Chiappe, Siegel, & Gottardo,

2002; Cummins, 1979). Molteno's approach was complex: they tended to take 2 to 3 years, produced formal curricula for the formal system in several languages, and, given the high cost of these activities, were largely funded by international donors or private philanthropies. Molteno also copyrighted all the materials it produced in order to recoup some of their development costs and to fund expansion into new areas. As a result, some African governments and donors found the materials too expensive and, despite successful pilots, did not continue with the approach (Letshabo, 2002; Lipson & Wixson, 2004).

Pratham Mobilizes Volunteers

Pratham (f. 1994),[15] an Indian NGO, began mobilizing citizen volunteers on a mass scale to conduct rapid reading and mathematics assessments of young children and to use the findings to move parents and communities to take action to improve levels of learning (Banerjee et al., 2007; Banerjee, Banerji, Duflo, Glennerster, & Khemani, 2008). Later, with funding from the Hewlett Foundation and others, Pratham helped Pakistan, Uganda, Kenya, and Tanzania to conduct household- and community-based surveys of children's reading ability. Pratham also hosted many visitors and provided technical assistance to early reading programs in other countries. In terms of its efforts to improve early learning, Pratham's remedial classes, mobile libraries, and tutors (*balsakhis*) operating after school hours all seemed to have more success than did efforts to introduce new learning materials or teaching approaches in formal classrooms. Pratham established great credibility among donors by allowing external researchers to evaluate its programs using RCTs and to publish the results, both favorable and less so. The scale of Pratham's work (its Annual Status of Education Review 2006 mobilized more than 20,000 volunteers) placed it in a category by itself in terms of implementation capacity.

BRAC Changes Its Curriculum

From 2004 to 2006 BRAC engaged linguists from an international NGO, SIL International (f. 1934), to help design new curricula for schools in indigenous communities in Bangladesh where Bangla was not the mother tongue. The experience changed BRAC's notion of what could be accomplished in early primary grades. With help from SIL, BRAC developed a new core Bangla language curriculum to teach reading and writing more systematically, placing more emphasis on children's oral skills and their ability to generate text. Ultimately, changing the reading curriculum led

BRAC to reorganize curricula in all subjects for Grades 1 and 2 in order to increase the time allocated to language from one to two 45-minute periods per day. The approach required many more books and materials, substantially increasing cost. All observers were so pleased by the results, however, that beginning in 2008 the new curriculum was scaled up into all Grade 1 and Grade 2 NFPE schools.

BRAC, with many capable curriculum developers on staff, most working in just one language, was probably an outlier in terms of how quickly EGR interventions could be designed and scaled up. Most African countries, like those served by Molteno, needed to take a multilingual approach to early language learning. For example, Malians speak 50 local languages, of which 13 are designated national languages, but, in order not to favor any of them, French is the official language. Developing curricula in at least 13 national languages for Grades 1 and 2 and designing a transition into an official language in later grades is expensive. Moreover, it calls for more linguists and curriculum developers than many ministries of education in sub-Saharan Africa or South and West Asia can muster.

Save Goes Extracurricular

Save the Children-U.S.[16] (f. 1934, Save) developed a labor-intensive, community-based approach to mother-tongue literacy learning and teaching materials. In the mid-1990s, it had adapted the BRAC NFPE model to some rural communities in Mali and Malawi where Save had long-established, intensive community development activities. In the late 1990s, Abigail Harris of Fordham University and a Harvard doctoral student, Amy Jo Dowd, supported by USAID, developed simple, largely oral mathematics and reading tests for Save's community schools in Malawi. Dowd subsequently developed the *Literacy Boost* program to:

- teach community members to make teaching and learning materials from local materials,
- train teachers to use those materials,
- establish extracurricular reading programs,
- encourage older children to read to their siblings, and
- persuade illiterate parents to encourage their children to read aloud to them.

The cost of locally available materials—dried beans, sticks, and so forth—was low, but the cost of organizing communities to undertake the activities and continue them involved much staff time, made possible by

Save's long-term commitment to the target communities. Save piloted *Literacy Boost* in Mozambique in 2009 and the next year started two new pilots in Nepal and Malawi. By the end of 2012 Literacy Boost was in 13 countries.[17] Like Molteno, Save had invested its own scarce internal development funds to design and test its approach and had to compete with other organizations for international donor funding. Save did not immediately place all its *Literacy Boost* materials in the public domain. Save also had concerns that other organizations might attempt to replicate this "low-cost" approach too quickly in new contexts without investing in the relatively expensive but critical adaptation work.

Other NGO Efforts in EGR

Other NGOs experimenting with early literacy improvement included PLAN International (f. 1937, PLAN)[18] in Niger and Mali and the Aga Khan Foundation (f. 1967, AKF) in Kenya and Tanzania. AKF also worked with CARE and other NGOs to implement reading improvement activities through the Partnership for Advancing Community Education in Afghanistan (f. 2006, PACE-A). The PACE-A case described in Figure 7.1 illustrates just a few of the difficulties of adapting and scaling up an innovation in a conflict zone. Other international NGOs such as SIL International and the Center for Applied Linguistics (f. 1959)[19] provided technical assistance to NGOs experimenting with multilingual instruction. Finally, the International Reading Association (f. 1956, IRA), a membership-based organization of educators, researchers, and policymakers in more than 100 countries, recruited members/experts to provide pro bono technical assistance for training, project design, and evaluation support in Third World countries.

Except for Pratham in India and BRAC in Bangladesh, most NGO efforts with EGR interventions, at least by 2012, were small-scale, and efforts to maximize their cost-effectiveness as they scaled up were ongoing. As described in Chapter 6, the preparation of appropriate teaching and learning materials for both students and teachers routinely costs more in funds, expertise, and time than most organizations can coax out of funders. In developing innovations for child survival, health NGOs and researchers in the global South were sometimes able to find longer-term funders, like the Rockefeller Foundation. Available funders for EGR in 2005 and 2006, however, such as the Hewlett Foundation, were largely committed to innovations that had already proven cost-effective in one context and were "ready to scale-up." Other, larger-scale donors, therefore, continued working with governments to promote whatever degree of innovation was possible in the process of expanding national systems of primary education.

Figure 7.1. Scaling Up Early Grades Reading and Mathematics Interventions: Partnership for Advancing Community Education in Afghanistan (PACE, 2006–2011)

The Partnership for Advancing Community Education in Afghanistan (PACE-A, f. 2006)* was one of the first efforts by an international NGO to apply EGRA and develop early grades reading interventions on a significant scale. PACE-A's experience illustrates a few of the complexities that "simple" reading programs tend to encounter in new and conflict-affected contexts. In Afghanistan, delivery agents—teacher trainers/field supervisors willing to live in the field and educated village residents willing to work for a meager and often irregular salary—were scarce. The target ratio for teachers to supervisor was 10:1 but in some areas it was 70:1. Neither firing nor hiring delivery agents based on purely on performance was always possible.

In 2006, the PACE-A monitoring and evaluation staff quickly developed a battery of tests for EGRA and similar Early Grades Mathematics tests in Dari and Pashto and used them to establish baseline levels of achievement. At the end of the 1st year, however, reading and mathematics results had not improved, at least in part because the existing textbooks and curriculum used in these schools did not cover the core components of reading. Project staff quickly designed supplemental teaching and learning materials and teacher training, but even without piloting, these materials did not reach the field until almost the end of the 2nd year. The training itself revealed that a few teachers themselves could not read fluently in the language of instruction. In addition, over time, security in some of the areas served by the project had deteriorated; monitoring and evaluation staff who a year earlier had accompanied and closely supervised the assessors could not do so for the second assessment. Not surprisingly, the second end-of-year assessment produced questionable results; the percentage of children who could read with understanding went from 54% to an improbable 94%. Nonetheless, as feedback came from the field about the strengths and weaknesses of the teaching and learning materials and of the teacher training, both were revised, but these revisions were not introduced in the field until late in the 3rd year.** Things take longer than expected.

*CARE-US, International Rescue Fund, Aga Khan Foundation, and Catholic Relief Services constituted the Partnership. The Partnership supported one-classroom community schools along the lines of BRAC primary schools as well as some more conventional, graded schools.

**This project was later the subject of a randomized controlled trial that was partially sponsored by the Poverty Lab but did not use EGRA as an outcome measure. See www.povertyactionlab.org/evaluation/effect-village-based-schools-evidence-rct-afghanistan

GOVERNMENT EFFORTS TO IMPROVE EARLY GRADES READING

Smaller donors like the Hewlett Foundation as well as larger donors such as USAID and the World Bank were looking for innovations that might have a large-scale impact before the MDG deadline in 2015. Reading activities had long been a modest part of foreign-donor support to some ministries of education. Nevertheless, RTI, the NGOs described above, and, increasingly, other organizations framed their EGR activities as something innovative and fundamental for EFA:

- EGRA as a quick yet potentially reliable leading indicator of education quality;
- a menu of high-quality EGR interventions, particularly relevant in primary schools with high levels of dropout;
- both grounded in some principles of cognitive science and interventions tested with RCTs; and
- leading to a discrete set of activities that could be accomplished in the time frame of most donor funding cycles and at least before 2015.

Some governments were galvanized by the results of EGRAs in their countries and began reforming their primary school curriculum almost immediately upon receiving results. This was the case in the Gambia, Nicaragua, Ethiopia, and Egypt. In other countries, including Senegal and Mali, where baseline EGRA findings were just as dismal as in Gambia, Nicaragua, Ethiopia, and Egypt, the data did not move government action in education onto a new trajectory.

RTI itself first ventured beyond measurement to pilot and compare several EGR interventions in formal government schools in Liberia. With Liberia still recovering from decades of civil war, the project had more leeway in shaping the curriculum and teacher training than might have been the case in other, more stable school systems. Support from both USAID (2008–11) and the World Bank enabled RTI to incorporate an RCT into the project from the start. The trial measured the relative impact of two treatments. In "light" treatment schools, researchers measured achievement in Grades 2 and 3, informed the community of the results, and provided assistance in community involvement. In "full" treatment schools, researchers did the same, but also trained teachers to assess student performance continuously and provided frequent school-based pedagogic support and additional resource materials and books. In the control schools, researchers simply measured achievement. A teacher kit with daily lesson plans focused on scope (what to teach), sequence (when to teach it), and an instructional model (how to teach). Combining the two grades in each group and comparing their baseline and final scores in November/December 2008 and May/June 2010, the no treatment (control group), light treatment, and full treatment groups increased their reading comprehension scores by 33%, 36%, and 130%, respectively. Although boys continued to perform better than girls in all reading tasks, girls gained more from the interventions than boys did.

By April 2010, before the pilot was complete, Liberian Ministry of Education officials were already talking about scaling up the program nationally. The pilot was relatively expensive, and the government had to make difficult decisions about which elements to scale back. According to teachers, principals, and instructional coaches surveyed at the end of the pilot, the program's most effective elements were, in order of importance: teacher training tied to clear and explicit lesson plans; coach support; and book materials, all expensive components. In contrast, the elements identified as least important—reading competitions, student report cards, radio shows, and school report cards—were also less expensive components, typically associated with low-cost accountability measures (Davidson & Hobbs, 2013; Davidson, Korda, & Collins, 2011).

INSTITUTIONALIZATION:
GROWING AN EARLY GRADES READING COMMUNITY OF PRACTICE

Many of the early adopters who were helping to diffuse EGR to various countries and organizations shared common eidetic experiences. Some had spent years working with or supporting others' work with community-based approaches. As a result, all were familiar with a short list of problems that dogged efforts to expand and improve primary schools in many of the countries with the farthest to go to achieve UPC, and perceived in EGR a promising approach to address many of them. Abadzi and Gove each had helped prepare country background papers for the highly critical 2006 primary education portfolio review for the World Bank. They recognized in EGR approaches several characteristics particularly well suited to what large, bureaucratic donors could fund and what governments with limited implementation capacity could manage:

- Able to produce quantitative results for a significant number of children within 3 to 5 years;
- Not dependent on systemwide reform or professionalization of teachers to succeed;
- Based on technical recommendations from credible academics;
- Making minimal demands for new or expensive technology; and
- Producing results readily understood by all stakeholders, from ministers to illiterate parents.

Several of the early EGRA adopters had studied the work of international research centers in other sectors, such as the International Maize and Wheat Improvement Center in Mexico and the International Center for

Diarrheal Disease Research in Bangladesh. They were familiar with use-oriented fundamental research and action research and were sympathetic to trial and error as an essential activity in scaling up. A significant number had earned doctoral degrees from major U.S. universities that encouraged their graduates to go out and shape future international education policy. All could give passionate examples of classrooms they had visited where children in their 3rd or 4th grade of elementary school could not read a single word in a sentence and where teachers welcomed programmed lessons that helped them to produce tangible improvements in student learning in a relatively short time.

Much of the early diffusion of EGRA and related interventions was, therefore, relational, based on the enthusiasm of these early adopters and others like them, their personal ties, and the networks they created as they moved from one organization to another in the normal course of their careers. None of the early adopters began as experts in reading, but they consciously set out to create a community of practice to identify and improve metrics, norms, and directions for the field. Their energy and interest in technology and quantitative analysis attracted many young professionals savvy in information and communication technology. For example, Save the Children created a fellows program for doctoral students in education who were interested in conducting use-oriented research on its *Literacy Boost* program. The graduates from this program constituted a new cohort of young specialists in early reading in developing countries as they fanned out to several international organizations and maintained contact with one another. The early adopters also recruited academic reading experts who were eager to put their approaches in new contexts and, familiar with the reading wars in the United States and United Kingdom, were prepared to handle pushback from other experts. After several years of assembling panels on early reading, in 2008 the number of Comparative and International Education Society (CIES) members involved in one or more of the EGR efforts created a critical mass for a Global Literacy Special Interest Group in CIES. The number of panels focusing on methods to measure and improve learning assessments at the CIES annual conference grew exponentially between 2004 and 2014. By 2010, the number of EGR-relevant reports funded by development agencies and organizations numbered in the hundreds. Peer-reviewed articles in journals with a large international readership, however, remained few (Abadzi, 2008; Abadzi et al., 2005). Journal articles were not a deliverable for USAID's EDDATA project, and others working under other funding mechanisms, such as Save's *Literacy Boost*, were just too busy.

Three-day EGR Community of Practice meetings in 2008 and 2010 each drew more than 180 participants from donor organizations, ministries of education, NGOs, universities, and research centers to discuss progress and setbacks, fine-tune their EGRA, and, in 2010, discuss their EGR intervention strategies. The meetings were sponsored by the largest donors to EGR activities, including the World Bank and USAID, and also benefited from contributions from smaller organizations, such as the Hewlett Foundation and RTI. The location of the meeting, just a block away from the Fast Track Initiative (FTI)[20] offices and professional ties between members of the community of practice meant that Robert Prouty, the FTI deputy director, later director (2011–2013), dropped in frequently, and he closed the 2008 workshop with 10 points he took away from the meeting, including:

- EFA targets for primary education are insufficiently precise, and insufficiently ambitious. . . . How about agreeing as an international community that we will seek to teach all children worldwide to read? That's a target to stir the blood, and one that's worthy of the billions of dollars we hope to inject into primary schools around the world. We need a global target.
- Some will argue that 60 wcpm by the end of Grade 2 is too reductionist. . . . [However,] 60 wcpm, or 80% of children reading with comprehension within two years, or something along those lines seems like a logical starting point to me, as we strive to shift the focus from access to learning. And there's nothing reductionist about that.
- We don't need more pilots to prove the point, but should be thinking from the beginning in terms of scaling up. How do we help countries design initiatives that may necessarily start small, but that are designed to go quickly to national scale as capacity is developed? (Transcript, Robert Prouty remarks to 2008 All Children Reading Community of Practice Meeting, World Bank)

The last statement may have unintentionally reinforced the common assumption that once an innovation is invented, it can be adapted and scaled up quickly within at least one country.

Community Growing Pains

The EGR approach did not proceed without pushback from several quarters, more often than not from those who did not share many of the early adopters' powerful experiences. Table 7.2 summarizes the technical claims and cautions from early adopters and critics about the components of EGR interventions. Some large-scale assessment experts based in the global North were justifiably concerned that EGRA would undermine efforts

Table 7.2. Early Grades Reading as New Education Goal: Claims and Cautions

EGR Characteristics	Claims	Cautions
Test		
Simple	Many teachers, government officials can do it	Easy to interpret fluency as speed alone
Replicable	Transparent template	Easily converted to a blueprint with rigid focus on phonics
Rigorous	Quantitative measure with good reliability	Scientific rigor, sophistication of large-scale written assessment remains more attractive to some
Fit for purpose	EGRA particularly useful in early grades, before children drop out	Framed as quicker, cheaper alternative to LS cross-national assessment but not cross-nationally comparable
Early benchmarking	Expect 100% of children can do it	Tendency to set benchmark too high: more than 30% of California 4th graders read below basic (NCES, 2013)
Compelling	Dramatic illustration of learning problem	Creates expectation that problem can be solved quickly
Predicts future achievement	Children who can read will learn more and perform better	May not prepare students well for conventional, rote-oriented exams that are highly valued by system and teacher
Tongue		
Harnessing mother tongue	Mother tongue instruction can improve and accelerate acquisition of reading in national language	Mother tongue instruction demands new mother tongue materials and, sometimes, additional teaching staff
Time		
Extra- and co- vs. curricular	Remedial, after-school programs are easier to implement and (therefore?) more effective	Children may not have time for chores
Deceptively . . .	Quick	Rate of progress slows as fluency increases?

185

Table 7.2. Early Grades Reading as New Education Goal: Claims and Cautions
(continued)

EGR Characteristics	Claims	Cautions
Text		
Deceptively . . .	Inexpensive teaching and learning materials	Inadequately funded
Quicker results, but teaching and learning materials don't appear overnight	Provides guidance and intervention in time period sufficient to keep kids from dropping out	Initial piloting of instruments and curriculum may take longer than 1 year
Learning to read more books	Children cannot memorize all classroom material	In addition to textbooks, children need many more leveled reading materials
Science vs. policy	Recent research in cognitive neuroscience aids legitimacy	Legitimacy challenged by recent failed efforts in U.K. & U.S. to push accountability reforms using early reading
Teach		
Easy	Inexperienced teachers like scripted approach	Experienced teachers may not follow scripted approach
Appropriate to delivery agents	Weak teachers can learn simple techniques: break reading instruction into small chunks, then ensure much practice and feedback to aggregate them	May not be able to implement effectively in school without changing teacher training, textbook, tongue, and/or time on task
Fit for purpose	Teachers can use EGRA to identify topics that need more work and students who need more help	Administrators and policy makers can "weaponize" EGR by establishing unrealistic goals for teachers and schools without the support necessary to achieve them
Pupil-teacher relations	EGRA can help individualize instruction, increase child-centered teaching	Difficult to implement in classrooms where pupil-teacher ratios are high. Slow learners may get stigmatized earlier.

Table 7.2. (continued)

EGR Characteristics	Claims	Cautions
Phonics vs. whole word	Systematic phonics is a well-known approach	May need more time for whole word instruction and early "text production" for second language/dialect learners.
Deceptively . . .	Simple	Requires behavior change. Teachers may need more in-class assistance to become systematic and sustain the changes.
Aides easy to train	Older children/ literate adults can become mentors/ tutors	Teachers need to learn how to manage aides effectively
Extracurricular	Currently, most effective programs in short-term are extracurricular. Even certified teachers do better outside classroom.	Teacher education needs to be reformed, curriculum needs to be reorganized to allow more time/systematic instruction in early grades for reading, & supervisors need retraining and doing more in-class mentoring
Social Mobilization		
Popularity	Good face value with all stakeholders at all levels	Stakeholders may value recitation or reading fluency as much as reading comprehension
Parents	Short list of actions for parents can lead to big improvement in scores	Mobilizing parents with low levels of literacy is very time-intensive.
Templates	Templates for social mobilization exist	May try to use social mobilization templates as blueprints
Donors	All donors interested in scalable innovations	No donors interested in funding trial-and-error, use-oriented research stage
International professionals	Selective global goal is more doable	Comprehensive global goals are institutionalized
Simple messages	Effective action for parents and teachers can be summarized in sound bites	Sound bites can over-promise

to integrate more Third World countries into existing cross-national tests, such as PIRLS, up to this time a growing niche industry. Those who championed education as a fundamental right for every child were also concerned, based on historical experience, that focusing on just one or two subjects in two or three grades would allow donors to shirk responsibility for funding the sort of "full" primary education, of good quality, envisioned in Dakar Goal 6. Furthermore, the EGR approach was simplistic compared with the more measured, nuanced approach to strengthening teachers promoted by the IRA. The two international staff at the IRA had limited presence in donor meetings. Within its limitations, however, IRA staff worked to introduce more teacher perspectives and less testing into the EGR approach. In addition, some academics saw parallels between the EGR approach and recent rigid approaches to teaching and testing early reading in the United States and the United Kingdom (Hoffman, 2012). Finally, critical scholars were concerned that the new foundations emerging from the capitalist North were, like their predecessor Rockefeller and Ford Foundations, pushing technical, palliative approaches that did not address fundamental economic and political reforms needed to break the cycle of poverty (Klees, 2012).

Internally, the Community of Practice itself had disputes. Several of RTI's competitors were surprised by the popularity of EGRA and, by extension, RTI among the donors. Some had played more central roles in USAID's earlier efforts to improve primary school instruction and had pioneered the use of rapid oral reading tests in several countries. In 2012, the head of a major RTI competitor quipped that USAID's education officers wanted "All RTI, all the time." In an article in a popular business magazine, an unidentified "USAID consultant" cited Crouch's serial assignments—from RTI, to the World Bank, to the Fast Track Initiative—as prima facie evidence of favoritism toward RTI by the Bank and FTI (Behar, 2012). In its defense, RTI pointed to the open-source EDDATA website, where it had made available all of its instruments, how-to manuals, and reports and the Early Grade Learning Community of Practice website, which RTI paid for out of its own development funds. The RTI staff also argued that other institutions were already using EGRA, or elements of it, without payment to RTI, and that RTI had in fact "trained up" others[21] who could perform the assessment at lower cost.

As discussed in Chapters 3 and 4, the international public health community did not immediately endorse ORS or its broad use. Indeed, research in later years changed fundamental notions about the formulation—sugar-based versus cereal-based versus homemade—and who could administer it and where. Similarly, the EGR community had internal debates, several dealing with the universality of methods. These were complicated by the involvement of several different subdisciplines—cognitive psychology, reading education, and linguistics—and the need to bring along the generalists who had entree to the donor organizations. Many of the reading researchers who initially became involved in the community were based in the English- or French-speaking worlds. But the spelling of those two languages—their orthographies—are among the most complex of any language. In contrast, in many of the countries with the farthest to go to achieve UPE, particularly in Africa, many languages have much simpler orthographies. Some psychologists, such as Share (2008) and Georgiou, Das, and Hayward (2008), argue that such languages can be taught—and tested—using fewer steps and subtasks than can English or French. Eventually, in 2011 the FTI funded an expert international panel to try to resolve these and other issues dealing with testing. As is the case with many scientific panels, all were not satisfied with the results. However, consistent with the panel's conclusions, most programs went ahead teaching the full range of components of reading and using a relatively large battery of tests routinely used for English. Research analyzing results of these programs and the tests they use could potentially resolve such debates (Abadzi, 2013). The panel did not endorse using any version of or subtest in EGRA as a universal measure. However, given that the limitations of short-term memory are universal, it is conceivable that some sort of cross-national comparisons could be developed in the future (Abadzi, 2012).

By 2010 the Community of Practice remained, therefore, a big tent, continuing to welcome all comers: mainly international development generalists, along with linguists, reading experts, and a smattering of psychologists. This community, therefore, did not constitute a cross-national group of scientists sharing common research methods, grounded in a common academic discipline like cognitive psychology, able to speak with one authoritative voice to policymakers. Several reports funded by donors and RTI at the end of the decade aimed, rather, to increase interest in and basic knowledge about EGR among more generalists and policymakers in the international development field (Gove & Cvelich, 2010; Roskos, Strickland, Haase, & Malik, 2009; Wagner, 2011). The back cover of the Gove and Cvelich edited volume (2010) listed dozens of organizations as members of the Community of Practice and contributors to the report.

The sum of these community-building activities bore fruit relatively quickly. All of the major donors featured EGR prominently in new education strategies issued from 2010 on: DfID (United Kingdom, 2010), USAID (United States, 2010), AusAID (Australia, 2011), the World Bank (2011), and the Global Partnership for Education (GPE, formerly FTI,

2012). USAID even went so far as to express its goals in time-bound, quantitative terms: 100 million children reading better by 2015. At the time these strategies were released, however, there were few large-scale EGR projects under way or universal, scientifically legitimated innovations on the shelf. Moreover, none of them were government-implemented or of sufficiently large scale to provide an empirical basis for estimating such numbers.

On the Way to 2015: Meetings and Papers

Between 2010 and the end of 2013, thousands of international experts and development professionals had participated in dozens of virtual and face-to-face meetings to discuss new post-2015 global development goals. Given that many education advocates had found the original formulation of the education MDGs unsatisfactory, post-2015 discussions offered an occasion to revise and make the new goals more compelling and worthy of global attention. Economists associated with the World Bank were among the first to call for a Millennium Learning Goal (Filmer, Hasan, & Pritchett, 2006).

Between 2006 and 2012 a series of forums and papers sponsored by organizations active in education for development explored how various indicators, including EGRA, might be used to track global progress on basic learning. For example, the Center for Universalizing Education at the Brookings Institution, with funding from the Hewlett Foundation and other donors, launched a *Global Compact on Learning* (f. 2011, Global Compact), asserting that lack of progress on EFA constituted a global crisis; that poor girls were often left behind, particularly in conflict areas; that better learning was a precondition to reducing poverty levels; and that learning, not access to schooling, would enhance individual abilities to lead healthier, more productive lives.

Under the rubric of the Global Compact, with funds from the Hewlett Foundation and other private-sector donors, the Center, UNESCO, and the UNESCO Institute of Statistics organized a Learning Metrics Task Force (f. 2011) that included dozens of other education-oriented donors and organizations. The Task Force set about developing universal domains and subdomains of competencies by level of schooling, preliminary to identifying common methods for measuring them and setting realistic global goals. A second task force was charged with cataloguing research priorities to support new efforts in learning. Both task forces advanced through a series of online exchanges and virtual and face-to-face meetings, and produced working papers by the end of 2012.

WORKING CONCLUSIONS

Largely dependent on education aid from Australia, DfID, USAID, and other large donors, EGR activities will rise and fall with the interest and budgets of those donors. In January 2014, USAID awarded a US$10 million, 5-year contract to a U.S. firm to take over the EGR Community of Practice work from RTI. Universal Research Corporation (URC) had significant prior experience with USAID projects in international health care quality assurance, communications, and social marketing projects. One of the seven components of the project includes:

> Filling the knowledge-practice gap by implementing research activities that result in the development, dissemination and accelerated uptake of early grade reading improvement methods.[22]

Nonetheless, EGRA's evolution through 2013 illustrates many of the generalizations posed in earlier chapters. By 2005, many education specialists in international development organizations were dissatisfied with the existing output measure for primary education: primary school completion. At that time, several international development professionals, many working in the education sector but not reading specialists, recognized in EGR something that would appeal to their major constituencies and would fit both the operational demands of the largest institutional donors and the pedagogical capacities of teachers in the weakest schools. By definition, therefore, the approach to EGRAs and interventions that emerged in the years following did not resemble what reading experts might have recommended. These international development professionals, however, quickly began recruiting academic reading experts and cognitive scientists to their cause, some of whom welcomed the opportunity to apply their work on a larger canvas. The professionals further increased the authority of their work by transforming what began as simple, informal oral reading tests, administered to opportunity samples,[23] into formal assessments that aspired to and often achieved high psychometric and sampling standards. Representative of these professionals, RTI International established new, higher standards for EGRA; developed an open-source toolkit for achieving those standards; and made results of all its assessments and related studies open-source, thus accelerating the spread of EGRA as a standard metric. All of this was abetted by the rise of the Internet and easy access to it.

Some of the similarities between the uses and weaknesses of EGRA and those of the Growth Monitoring component of the Child Survival initiative are indeed striking. Neither can improve the education or health status of a single child. Both require the identification and promotion of low-cost, simple interventions that have direct impact on children's welfare. Many of the interventions that held promise for improving early reading and early physical growth were developed by nongovernmental organizations (NGOs), for the most part on a small scale and often outside the formal government school and health systems, and few had been rigorously evaluated.

Nonetheless, the data that the early reading and Child Survival advocates generated attracted donor attention. In the education sector, some leading donors incorporated EGR into their education strategies and quickly began to encourage national governments to adapt, pilot, and scale-up some of these interventions. Meanwhile a Community of Practice was established, which continues to experience both competition and substantive differences, and research opportunities attracted a new generation of quantitatively oriented doctoral students into the subsector. Only 7 years after the first international development-oriented early reading papers began circulation in the field, EGR for non-Anglophone/Francophone languages is not yet institutionalized in international education doctoral programs and journals and specialized positions in international organizations, but it still might be. There was much individual agency at work here and, at the same time, much enacting of professional identity in the international development field and many references to models of reality, scripts, and blueprints. Abadzi used timed, 1-minute oral reading fluency tests to quantify widespread decoupling between the formal primary education system and what was happening in schools supported by international development donors. She was joined by a dozen or so professionals who saw themselves as actors authorized to help countries make a measurable impact on progress toward national and global goals. These professionals, consistent with norms in the international development, did not perceive themselves as creating and pressing external standards on unwilling countries. Many of them had encountered teachers in the most difficult contexts who welcomed the new approach and put it to good use. At the other end of the spectrum, both ministries and donors were intrigued by the potential of this new, apparently simple measure of primary education quality, with the potential to more tightly couple goals in the National Education Plan to performance at the classroom level. In many systems, however, the response to tighter coupling is new and different types of loose coupling. Hence it is by no means certain that tighter coupling will necessarily lead to the system improvement that promoters predict.

It is too early to conduct a meta-analysis of the EGR programs that are now under way in scores of countries. The degree of country ownership for early reading as a national goal varies greatly across the countries that have accepted donor funds for this purpose. Energetic acceptance of the measure and its reform implications has occurred where there was leadership, and appears to have lagged where it was handled through routine ministry channels. Although EGRA might be a smaller, quicker, cheaper assessment, the early reading activities prescribed to improve achievement demanded profound changes in the standard operating procedures of most conventional primary school systems. Despite its simple appearance, the EGR approach demands changes in textbooks, teacher pre- and inservice training, and allocation of classroom time in at least two grades. This approach also demands a change in the definition of education achievement and in assessment procedures.

Between 2010 and 2012, however, only a few early reading interventions were ready for RCTs, and none were universally applicable in all languages. No systematic fundamental use-oriented reading research was being done in international centers based in the global South; the Gates and Hewlett Foundations were not underwriting the long-term investments in international education research that the Rockefeller and Ford Foundations had financed in health and agriculture research from the 1960s through the 1980s. National centers in the global North indeed were conducting some action research relevant to the global South, but Northern-devised innovations needed experienced reading experts to carry and adapt them to the South. For example, RTI International recruited Sandra Hollingsworth to help national educators adapt the Systematic Methods for Reading Success she had developed at the University of California, Berkeley, for use in South Africa and Mali (Hollingsworth & Gains, 2009). The length of her tenure in both places, however, was short, and neither government provided support for further adaptation during scale-up. Once such an intervention was successful in one language, however, many countries still lacked trained curriculum developers who could adapt—not just translate—the prescribed improved teaching and learning materials into other languages.

The strategies of several major donors, including USAID and the GPE, nonetheless assumed that, having identified the gap in early literacy, interventions to close the gap could be quickly developed and scaled up. Between 2008 and the first quarter of 2014, USAID alone launched at least 25 3-to-5-year projects worth about US$700 million, including some countries with ongoing or recent conflict. In light of the cases examined in the last three chapters, the relatively short time frame of these strategies and projects is insufficient. If donors demand systemic or systemwide results (as opposed to project-level results) measured on international metrics within 3 to 5 years, the most likely result will be Hirschman's *fracaso*-mania described in Chapter 4, a rush to declare failure too quickly.

Alternatively, these projects and, more important, attempts to scale-up what is learned by them, can explicitly or implicitly clarify some of the factors set forth in earlier chapters, particularly those relating to the role of organizations, the nature of innovations, and the role of environment or context. For example, these projects can test whether conducting field experiments and small pilots followed by large pilots before going to scale-up, using trial and error, must take as much time per context as the BRAC cases suggest. The primary education sector in the international development field is not so flush with promising innovations that it can afford to dismiss any too easily or to scale them up on the strength of good pilot studies alone, only to have them crash and burn. Good social scientists learn more from incremental failures than from instant success, and good development professionals know that almost anything is better than starting from scratch.

CHAPTER 8

Conclusions

Why Compare?

It is the increasing economic importance of human capital, consisting of the acquired abilities of people—their education, work experience, skills, and health—that explains most of modern economic progress.

—Theodore Schultz (1993)

Both health and education are key to modern notions of national and individual prosperity. Global goals such as Health for All and Education for All represent efforts by international development organizations to hold governments accountable for their unprecedented global commitments to economic and social progress for all citizens. In the process, by intent or not, these organizations impose some small measure of rational governance at the global level.

The foundations for these goals lie in the various declarations of and covenants pertaining to human rights deriving from the Universal Declaration of Human Rights (1948) and codified in the International Covenants of Civil and Political Rights and of Economic, Social, and Cultural Rights (ESCR), promulgated at the height of the Cold War. These covenants embody two notions that have roots in several cultures but clearly express core Western Enlightenment values: first, that educated individuals—distinct from earlier families or tribes—are the building blocks of modern nation-states, and second, that rationality, justice, and equity form core organizing principles for governance in and of such states. Neither notion has ever been fully implemented, but they remain powerful scripts for rallying and mobilizing global action now, well into the 21st century. Almost all nation-states acceded to these covenants within a decade of their promulgation, for a variety of reasons, only one of which was whole-hearted embrace of Western Enlightenment culture. Particularly in the global South, far from the heartland of the Western Enlightenment, nation-states sought to appease the powerful combatants in the Cold War, build partnerships with future investors and aid donors, and join the community of modern nation-states.

As a result, in many countries, adherence to global commitments like the ESCR Covenant was only loosely coupled to financial, political, technical, and implementation capacity and resources at the national and local levels.

The case studies assembled in Chapters 2 through 7 aim to uncover some of the mechanisms by which international development organizations try to tighten coupling between commitments to the ESCR Covenant and what nation-states actually do. The mechanisms include:

- sector-specific global conferences and declarations that issue . . .
- time-bound targets at the global level that translate into . . .
- national plans of action that are monitored by adopting . . .
- cross-nationally comparable indicators to be used for . . .
- advocacy campaigns at the global and national levels demanding . . .
- innovations that can provide better services, more quickly delivered to all citizens, regardless of their gender, location, ethnicity, or other collective identification.

In 2000, goals in a dozen sectors, many of them promulgated using these mechanisms, were consolidated into a list of six Millennium Development Goals.

The current world model of mass primary education predates the ESCR Covenant and has a firm hold on the imaginations of all the organizations, professionals, and bureaucrats crafting and designing activities to realize the universal right to education promised in the covenant. This model links the notion of mass schooling with the socialization of children into citizens. Within the model, governments are expected to play a dominant role in providing mass schooling, and they in turn expect to play a major role in directing these schools. The theory of human capital may assume a close link between individual education and national development. Nonetheless, in the development field, donors and recipient governments appear to agree that a lack of primary schooling is not a life-threatening condition and, therefore, does not merit stopgap measures that would deviate from the world model. This model has a dampening effect on innovation in primary education, particularly in comparison with innovation in other sectors, such as health.

WHY TWO SECTORS?

Many analyses of progress toward global education goals impute to the education sector and to national interests obstacles that are in fact common to efforts to promote global goals in any sector. Figure 8.1 revisits several

Figure 8.1. The Relevance of World Culture to Global Goals

G2.1. Global initiatives that can be associated with prior formal commitments made at the global level, by many nation-states, gain legitimacy somewhat independent of the means to achieve them.

G2.2. Loose coupling between global goals and national/local actions will vary inversely with the degree of connection between a specific context and its participation in or contact with the Western Enlightenment.

G2.3. Over time, demand for nation-states to conform to international commitments to global goals will increase and the means for quantitatively tracking those commitments will multiply and become standardized.

G2.4. As more global initiatives are launched, a blueprint for global conferences/declarations/goals/global monitoring emerges, enabling new global initiatives to launch more quickly than older ones did.

G2.5. As the identity of the modern, internationalist, humanitarian leader and of the international development professional becomes established, champions for new global initiatives take less time to establish themselves.

G2.6. Successful scripts for promoting global initiatives will incorporate key world culture themes: equity (rights-based), material well-being (technical efficiency), and individualism (for all, humanitarian universalism).

general generalizations about global initiatives derived from the comparison of Health for All (HFA) and Education for All (EFA) initiatives in Chapter 2.

These generalizations provide a jumping-off point for other observations at various levels in later chapters, including the following questionable tendencies on the part of development professionals:

- generalizing across sectors, irrespective of variations in the scientific foundations, complexity, and state mandates underlying them;
- neglecting to fund use-oriented research relevant to Third World countries;
- defining innovations in terms of discrete deliverables, without adequate attention to delivery agents or delivery support systems;
- relying on nongovernmental organizations (NGOs) to produce innovations and expecting governments to scale them up;
- underestimating the tension between government and NGOs created by world models and blueprints;
- failing to perceive the mismatch between the relatively short time frame of conventional donor project cycles versus the time necessary for effective innovation and diffusion;
- confusing contexts with countries and underestimating the time necessary to adapt and scale-up an innovation in each new context;

- fragmenting nuanced, comprehensive approaches into simplistic, selective ones;
- demanding sustainable systems and institutions faster than historical precedent justifies; and
- burying failures instead of learning from them.

In the course of gathering material for this book, I came across many health professionals who were strongly convinced of the multiplier effects of education on health interventions and eager to work more closely with education researchers. From the point of view of education researchers, health research sites and databases have much to offer. In Bangladesh, for example, the Health and Demographic Surveillance System at Matlab has collected data for over 40 years for a population of some 225,000 in 142 villages every 2 months. The data cover births, deaths, marriages, divorces, migration, internal movement, and household splits, and periodic surveys collect additional data on occupations and household assets. Given that one of the perennial problems of education research is controlling for the socioeconomic background of children and their families, such a site could be a boon to education researchers. The Institutional Review Board at the Diarrhea Center applies rigorous, up-to-date ethical oversight for all types of research at Matlab, from anthropological participant observation through field trials for cholera vaccines. The board has already reviewed and approved several small studies of preprimary education interventions.

WHY ORGANIZE?

"Let's get this thing organized!" is a quintessential modern rallying cry. The tendencies listed above are not unique to international development organizations, and as such, they do not necessarily indicate inordinate amounts of willful ignorance or desire for control. Rather, they are typical of organizations in fields where inputs and production processes are not standardized. Outputs and outcomes are difficult to measure in real time and dollars, and funding is not commensurate with mandates. Under such conditions, organizations tend to adopt common frames, models, blueprints, and norms that may be only loosely coupled to historical precedent, organizational capacity, or measurable results. After more than 50 years of this sort of formalization and standardization, some of the older organizations in the international development field are approaching Max Weber's "iron cage" stage, where the multiplication of highly rationalized rules and standard operating procedures leaves little room for independent or innovative action. This has ripple effects throughout the field, as younger, less formal organizations may be obliged to adopt more rigid standard operating procedures to the extent that they are dependent for resources on older organizations. Professionals in international development organizations sometimes moan about rigid Third World bureaucrats, but the pot may be calling the kettle black.

Most meta-analyses of innovation tend to miss the organizational level of analysis, focusing instead on politics, individual leadership, contextual factors, or characteristics of the innovation. In many cases, however, organizations are the crux of the issue. With the right organization, a leader can accomplish unbelievable feats on a global level; with no organization, very little is accomplished. Figure 8.2 summarizes some of the organizational characteristics that aid in launching and sustaining global initiatives and other characteristics that aid in diffusing innovations linked to those initiatives to new contexts. For the former, this calls for funding organizations, often international angel investors, and some contexts already using low-cost

---

Figure 8.2. Organizational Factors That Aid in . . .

. . . launching and sustaining global initiatives

O2.1. Funding organizations support at least some components of the initiative.

O2.2. Local organizations in some of the contexts with the farthest to go to meet the goals of the global initiative, have:

- piloted innovations relevant to some part of the initiative and established some as cost-effective and
- a mandate to act and are headed by one or more charismatic, competent innovators or leaders.

O2.3. Angel investors stand ready to support the early invention, adaptation, and piloting of new innovations.

O2.4. The initiative does not demand profound changes in culture and/or standard operating procedures in either implementing or funding organizations.

. . . diffusing innovations linked to global initiatives to new contexts

O5.2. An *organization*—governmental or nongovernmental—has previously demonstrated its ability to deliver services effectively to the target context or a similar one.

    O5.2.1. The organization has demonstrated its *capacity to learn by trial and error.*

    O5.2.2. The organization has identified *potential delivery agents in the target context.*

    O5.2.3. If it is not the implementer, *the government* supports the channeling of donor funds to an alternative implementer, such as an NGO.

    O5.2.4. *The donor* tolerates trial and error well.

        O5.2.4.1. The innovation can demonstrate effectiveness within the *funding cycle of the donor.*

innovations that support global initiatives. In many contexts, the prerequisite innovations have been developed by NGOs on a small scale. Many more contexts, however, lack the right combination of organizations—governmental or nongovernmental, national or international—with the characteristics prerequisite to scaling up quickly. This should not suggest that it will be impossible to scale-up in difficult contexts, only that it will cost more and take more time than it might in a context where capable organizations are already at work.

In Chapters 5 and 6, several governments resisted offers by international development organizations to scale-up unconventional NGO programs in primary health in the 1980s and in primary education in the 1990s. Underfunded ministries will be inclined to use the primary education system to establish more control over basic service delivery at the grass roots and to ensure that the maximum amount of donor funds flows through government channels. Even where government organizations are already working in the target context and ready to work with NGO innovations, government bureaucrats may not have the right combination of skills and/or the flexibility necessary to adapt an innovation piloted on a small scale to large-scale implementation. Finally, with the passage of each decade, donor and government organizations become more rigid. In Bangladesh, rolling out a decade after OTEP, NFPE faced not just more rigid international donors, but also more rigid national bureaucrats and politicians.

This is a conundrum: in most countries with the farthest to go to achieve global goals, governments are unlikely to have the flexibility and reach into underserved areas prerequisite to delivering a full primary education or basic health care, of good quality, to all children. But where NGOs do have those capabilities, they may not be allowed. In Bangladesh, formal schools were more consistent with the world model of mass education than NFPE, and this added authority to the government's case. If the government had pursued something other than that model—for example, had instituted a purely religious education in *madrassahs* that did not include reading and writing instruction in the vernacular—the response of the international development community might well have been different.

Finally, the role of private philanthropic organizations has also changed over time. However much they may be criticized for supporting capitalist imperialism, older foundations—Ford, Rockefeller—once served as patient investors for tropical laboratory and clinical research as well as field trials and pilots in the Western scientific tradition. Newer foundations—Gates, Hewlett—seem as impatient for results as older international development organizations are. The likelihood that babies are going out with the bathwater has only increased as more rigid accountability mechanisms spread. A recent round of foundation grants called for NGOs based in the Third

World to scale-up reading innovations in new contexts that had previously not been tested in more than one context. A meta-analysis of the individually contracted and designed evaluations for these grants, conducted after only 3 years, not surprisingly, found little impact (McEwan, 2013).

WHY PROFESSIONALS?

The professionals who move between large international development organizations to staff foundations' international departments are the main carriers of this impatience. They carry with them, from organization to organization, both a culture specific to the international development field and rationalizations for the rigidities of multiple former employers. Like all professionals, they have scripts and identities, one of which demands that they exercise agency in order to improve economic and social conditions in the countries to which they are assigned.

Like proverbial frogs in a pot of water put on to boil, however, some of them have not noticed the increasing gap between their professional ideals and the increasing formalization and rigidity of the leading organizations in the field. As a result, many remain convinced that their organizations can support the development process for innovations. They do not recognize the mismatch between the trial-and-error approach and their organization's operating procedures and the limitations on their own professional agency.

Champions of global goals like Mahler and Grant arose from the ranks of development professionals, but they came to their positions with much time in the field, much more experience with trial and error. Since then, international development as an organizational field has become more formalized. Today's development professionals are likely to have spent less time in the field, more in specialized higher education and in inservice training in their own organizations, and be more committed to various development theories than Mahler or Grant ever were.

Development professionals today, however, have a great arena for action that was not available in Mahler and Grant's day. New communication technology—radio, television, film at the time—helped to revolutionize social mobilization and made a major contribution to Child Survival. Today another generation of information and communication technology (ICT)—computers, the Internet, tablets, and smartphones—has helped education professionals develop an epistemic community that has marshaled a case for a new, more selective approach to EFA that has influenced the education strategies of some of the largest international donors. Whether that community can now find more flexible funding to identify and support innovation to support those strategies is being played out now.

WHY INNOVATE?

The modern world is enamored of the new, that is, of innovation. Indeed, as the cases in this book illustrate, the previously unreached contexts that universal goals intend to enter need new approaches, even for something as "universal" as ORT. Adams and Chen (1981) argued that the initial acceptance of an innovation will be greater where the difference between the innovation and the status quo is minimized. Indeed, many mothers find traditional carrot and chicken soup, made with a more precise recipe, a more appealing type of ORT than some powder sprinkled into cold water. The many differences between NFPE and formal schools made NFPE less, not more, appealing to bureaucrats in Bangladesh.

In contrast, development professionals, educated and living largely in the Western world, tend to be more enamored of innovations that are dramatically different from the status quo. For example, development organizations have invested significant resources in innovative uses of information and communication technology (ICT), but these have proven much more successful in improving monitoring and in social mobilization than they have in instruction. As of late 2013 the Poverty Lab had conducted multiple studies on ICTs in education and found none of them cost-effective. In 2012, USAID, Australian aid, and World Vision pooled funds and issued a "Grand Challenge for Development: All Children Reading" that called for proposals using ICTs to improve the quality of reading instruction. The revolution in education quality through ICTs in the First World, however, has been heralded at least once a decade since World War II and has yet to arrive. It remains to be seen whether the new Third World knockoffs of expensive hardware like tablet computers will reduce the price sufficiently to get this revolution going in the Third World.

Figure 8.3 summarizes some of the factors of innovations identified in Chapters 2, 5, and 6 that aid in launching and sustaining global initiatives and speed their diffusion to new contexts.

This list is itself no innovation but tracks closely with the factors identified in many earlier analyses of innovations in education in the Third World (Adams & Chen, 1981; Fullan, 1989; Havelock & Huberman, 1978). The issue for many in the development field, therefore, is not what kind of innovations we need but how to support the creation of more effective ones. Each of these writers warned of the need to learn from failure and the temptation to toss an innovation aside too soon. Most agree that small organizations and visionary individuals provide better incubators for young innovations than government programs. Chapters 5 and 6 also produced several characteristics of contexts that aid in the process of scaling up innovations.

Figure 8.3. Characteristics of Innovations That Aid in the Process of . . .

. . . launching and sustaining global initiatives

In at least one context, innovation(s) exist that are:

I2.1. salient to the initiatives,

I2.2. simple,

I2.3. stand-alone,

I2.4. cheap to produce and deliver,

I2.5. in the public domain,

I2.6. do not demand unprecedented levels of sustained behavior change,

I2.7. amenable to social mobilization,

I2.8. produce results quickly,

I2.9. produce results that are dramatic, evident to the naked eye,

I2.10. validated with quick, cheap, universal outcome indicator(s), and

I2.11. authorized as universal by high science.

. . . diffusing global initiatives to new contexts

For each new context, innovations exist that have been:

I5.1.1. tested and evaluated in a context similar to the new context,

I5.1.2. piloted by delivery agents available in the new context,

I5.1.3. championed by at least one group with legitimacy in the international
    scientific community, and

I5.1.4. rationalized in terms of quantitative outcome measures that have face
    validity with donors, politicians, and the target group.

The modern fascination with universality has been a stumbling block in scaling up many innovations. Historically, donors have been loath to fund two-track approaches, simultaneously supporting one strategy to address the stopgap needs of students currently falling out of the mainstream system and another to address the long-term need to reform and strengthen that system. This reluctance may be changing. In Bangladesh and perhaps some other countries, major donors fund both the government's mainstream system and NGO-run alternative schools for working, language-minority, sexually abused, and older children. Sustaining this policy is complicated because innovations to reach and address the needs of marginalized children in smaller contexts are usually more expensive than innovations tested and ready to plug into nationwide school systems. Moreover, the notion of spending more on marginalized children than on mainstream children is a difficult one for governments everywhere.

Finally, there is the chicken-and-egg problem. The OTEP case demonstrates what can be done under extremely difficult circumstances with the right sense of urgency, a well-adapted innovation, and a scientifically authorized outcome measure. In contrast, NFPE was an innovation in search of a scientifically authorized outcome measure and EGRA was a scientifically authorized outcome measure in search of some relevant innovations. If, in the next decade or so, cognitive science were to establish universal ranges of cognitive stunting to which, absent quality learning activities, young children are subject, perhaps a greater sense of urgency might be generated for universal early and primary education. But could even evidence of stunting on a massive scale overcome the inertia of the current global model of mass schooling and the reluctance to take alternative stopgap measures to address its shortcomings?

WHAT ABOUT SCIENCE?

Professional norms and practices around innovation demand skeptical scrutiny, and so do putatively scientific ones. Much of the practice of normal science in each generation builds on principles that later generations will disprove or simply reject. Scientists whom later generations would label geniuses—Copernicus, Galileo, Newton—in their own time subscribed to many of those principles (Kuhn, 1962/1996). The problem with the principles in each generation was not so much that they were entirely false but that they were applied too broadly. For example, bloodletting, using leeches, had been widely prescribed for millennia for a head-spinning range of complaints. Modern medicine dismissed both bloodletting and leeches until the 1980s, when leeches were put back to work for very specific tasks, such as skin grafting.

The history of science suggests that it behooves each field in every generation to interrogate the science supposedly undergirding its most cherished presuppositions and rationalizations. Clearly the international development field—in which most education for development work is embedded—has overextended several assumptions. The reification of abstract, explicit knowledge leads us to ignore less systematic, more implicit knowledge, to value RCTs over trial-and-error action research. A narrow focus on individuals and human agency can lead to a neglect of the ways that organizations constrain the repertoire of action and the field of vision for individuals in them. The reification of free markets distracts us from recognizing how frequently the preconditions for free markets do not pertain, that resource dependency, professional jurisdiction, and—when all else fails—simple mimicry may explain the course of many organizations and projects. The reification of leadership in the modern world leads us to overlook the work of bureaucrats, professionals, and the pull of institutionalized routines and norms. The notion of universality has blinded us to the fact that education research in the First World has lost interest in critical issues confronting Third World school systems and that some investment in research embedded in the Third World is in order. The reification of quantitative data leads to the privileging of big data and the forgetting of its extremely shaky sources, particularly in the countries with the farthest to go to meet global goals.

One particularly insidious leech is the notion of sustainability. Sustainability began appearing in the international development discourse in the 1980s. In the name of sustainability, the structural adjustment approach encouraged borrower countries to reduce "bloated" bureaucracies by reducing the number of civil servants, in some cases including schoolteachers, and reducing or freezing salaries for those who remained, even as inflation rates soared. These policies effectively forced many teachers to look for second and third jobs to supplement their inadequate salaries. More recently, when donors encouraged governments to make primary education compulsory, to eliminate school fees, and in some cases, as in Bangladesh, to use stipends to increase enrollments, millions of new students were welcomed to primary school by dispirited teachers, many effectively absent while on duty.

Also in the name of sustainability, for several decades some of the largest donors refused to supplement primary school teacher salaries in the Third World. At the same time, they urged Third World governments there to look for ways to "recover costs" from students' families. However rational these concerns with sustainability, they ran directly contrary to historical precedent in most donor countries. In what country have illiterate parents in the bottom two deciles of the income distribution ever covered a significant part of the cost of educating first-generation learners in modern primary schools? BRAC has a better track record than most governments for recovering pennies from some of the most impoverished people in the world for some of the most prosaic services, for example, vaccinating chickens. What does it mean when this same organization concludes that cost recovery for primary schools for those same impoverished people is not cost-effective?

Science also warns us that quantity often changes quality. Lessons learned in a pilot or small-scale project may not apply to larger-scale efforts in the very same context. For example, engineers warn that even the supposedly immutable laws of physics may not apply to concrete in the unprecedented size of the structures used to construct the Three Gorges Dam in China. Consider also NFPE, working on an unprecedented scale in Bangladesh, with no empirical precedents for what would and would not work. Yet with jaw-dropping hubris, expatriate consultants insisted that NFPE must pay their teachers more or must incorporate Western-style, activity-based, child-centered teaching, regardless of the capacities of the candidates for Program Officer and the paraprofessional teachers available in rural Bangladesh.

WHAT IS TO BE LEARNED?

The sociology of organizations community debates whether old organizations can learn or whether certifiably innovative approaches will emerge principally from new organizations. Most large donors to education in developing countries like to think of themselves as learning organizations that incorporate into their work some lessons from the education sector and management literature in First World countries, as well as other lessons from monitoring and evaluating the projects they themselves fund. These lessons, however, are better characterized as potential factors that await empirical data to confirm or disprove them.

Much of the education research relevant to the countries with the farthest to go to meet the MDGs is currently being produced by development organizations. The 3- to 5-year project cycle typical in those organizations rarely provides an opportunity to follow up promising findings (or failures!) with systematic research. When funding ends for one project, organizations must move on to the next project, which will generate its own idiosyncratic lessons—lessons learned in a particular sector, in a particular context, at a particular time, within the scope of particular innovations, implemented with more or less integrity, within specific funding constraints. Research that is conducted to monitor and evaluate educational development projects, therefore, can inform decisions about specific approaches in specific contexts, and its dissemination may spark the imagination of others to adapt something similar in another context. But it rarely allows education researchers to build on one another's work and advance research methods and knowledge in the field to the extent that health researchers regularly do.

Somewhat independent of development donor funding, the Abdul Latif Jameel Poverty Action Lab (f. 2005, J-PAL) continues to conduct research and compile data to analyze the cost-effectiveness of stand-alone education interventions in Third World schools on student learning. For example, based on an analysis of randomized controlled studies in nine African and Asian countries of varying size and complexity, the interventions that result in the biggest increase in test scores per US$100 invested were providing earnings information (Madagascar), contract teachers (Kenya), tracking students' achievement levels (Kenya), and increasing the legitimacy and authority of the school committee (Indonesia).[1] However, these were relative successes; we do not know the limits of each intervention. Does the impact of the intervention vary based on the stage in the literacy acquisition process? Are some interventions more useful than others at the beginning of that process? Which of these interventions can help children acquire the later stages of literacy acquisition, including reading with comprehension? Where is the notion of "dosage," so important in health research? In early reading, for example, how much effort, for how long, with what frequency, and what type and amount of materials and human resources could consistently ensure that the average child would read fluently with comprehension by Grade 3 or 4? In health sector terms, therefore, early grade reading interventions lack both a universal formula (or a menu of potential interventions) and effective dosage protocols. Without that formula or those protocols, there can be no price tag, and without an "unconscionably low" price tag, there will be no shaming of the First World into paying for it.

The Child Survival case suggests that education professionals and academics should not be ashamed that we have little immutable science that can be brought to the aid of global goals in education. Science in other sectors is often shakier than we think. However, we are culpable, given the agency expectations built into our roles in society, for failing to establish research institutes where they are needed the most, institutes funded not by development donors, but by longer-term, less intrusive sources, with more world-class technical oversight than individual projects can provide. Ideas for how to go about this may be stimulated by visits to research centers like the Diarrhea Center or to members of the Consultative Group for International Agricultural Research. Without founding a new research center, education research might be carried out under the oversight and in the enumerated field sites of international research centers in other sectors. Meanwhile, much can be learned from all sorts of education research currently under way, even if such research does not produce the innovations we would like as fast as we would like.

Are we learning more from very expensive RCTs than we did from all those case studies of education in developing countries that international organizations have been compiling since the 1970s and more recent collections on project and organizational websites? Like the earlier case studies, the J-PAL findings do not offer blueprints to be replicated in other contexts. Rather, they invite professionals to learn more and may inspire adaptation in new contexts. Like the more recent websites such as EDDATA, the advantages of the J-PAL studies, therefore, lie chiefly in careful statements of their methods and the quantification of their findings, increasing the likelihood that other researchers in other contexts will build on their work. The disadvantages are that donor organizations will privilege quantitative studies over other types of research that may tell us what factors we might want to study in the future and why.

Given the fixation on innovations in the international development field, new databases of education innovations, such as the DfID-funded Center for Education Innovations at Results for Development or the IIEP's Planning for Improved Learning, as well as earlier databases and collections of primary education innovations developed by UNESCO, cry out for both quantitative and qualitative analyses. It is to be hoped that one or more such analyses would pay some attention not just to deliverables, but also to the alignment of delivery agents and delivery support services, and the role of different types of organizations. Figure 8.4 lists a few of the contextual factors identified in Chapters 5 and 6 that we expect come into play in such comparative analyses.

WHAT WILL IT COST?

The Millennium Development Goals were in large part an effort to identify big achievements that could be accomplished with relatively small amounts of money within historically established trajectories (Vandemoortele, 2011). J-PAL efforts to account for cost and test cost-effectiveness are the most recent manifestation of a decade of fitful efforts to establish that global education goals can be met for a cost acceptable to international donors. This is because almost all studies find a significant shortfall between the amount countries with the farthest to go to achieve the goals are willing and able to pay, and the expected cost of achieving universal primary education. The

Figure 8.4. Characteristics of Contexts That Aid in the Process of Scaling Up Innovations

---

C5.3. The *size of the population* in the target context—an area unified by a common language, culture, livelihoods, and social structure—*justifies the cost* of initial adaptation, field trials, and pilots of the deliverable, delivery agents, and delivery support services.

C5.4. Within the target context, sufficient delivery sites are relatively *free from internal conflict*.

C5.5. A prior intervention has achieved similar levels and types of *community participation* within the target context.

C5.6. Delivery agent functions—e.g., teachers, POs, subdistrict and district supervisors—can be adapted to *labor available* at or willing to relocate to the delivery sites.

    C5.6.1. An acceptable level of commitment and diligence on the part of delivery agents can be attained through some combination of salaries, performance incentives, and/or moral suasion.

C6.1. Managers/experts who have hands-on experience scaling up an innovation in one context are willing to take up residence and assist with the adaptation and scaling up of that innovation in another context.

C6.2. The target context or a significant number of delivery sites are relatively free from external conflict.

---

international community, therefore, must be persuaded to fill in the short-fall. Delamonica, Mehrotra, and Vandemoortele (2004) estimated that the global shortfall in primary education for 2001 to 2015 was approximately 11% of what developing countries currently spend on education, with approximately 60% of the global shortfall occurring in sub-Saharan Africa and South Asia. The authors concluded, "Education for All is affordable at the global level. Compared with the expected economic benefit, it is clearly an excellent investment opportunity" (p. 20). Five years later, Glewwe and Zhao (2006), however, reviewed four existing cost projections and concluded that until the primary education subsector established which policies or activities could achieve the education MDG, Universal Primary Education, no one could estimate the cost.

Persuading governments and donors to make large investments today to reap large rewards later is harder than persuading them to make smaller investments today for moderate rewards later. Hence the search for what Kenneth King called the Golden Fleece of low-cost quality education for all (1991) and for the low-cost innovations for primary education that can make it happen. As school systems move closer to universal enrollment, the cost per child of enrolling the last 5 to 10% in primary school is likely to be much higher than the same cost for the 90 to 95% of children already enrolled.

In these efforts, all donor funds are not equal. Paradoxically, those driven by the security interests of the West were, in earlier generations, some of the more generous and flexible. Cold War interest in shoring up SEATO launched the Cholera Lab in the 1960s; population control concerns pressed for additional funding for maternal-child health and girls' education since the 1970s; and since 2001, War on Terrorism concerns helped to allocate historically unprecedented amounts of funding for primary education programs in Muslim countries. As more of these funds were channeled through highly formalized bilateral aid organizations, however, the monitoring became more rigid. Hence the case study of PACE-A (see Figure 7.1 on page 180). Informants from the early years of the Cholera Lab uniformly asserted that the amount and type of research they were able to do in the 1960s would not be possible under today's much more detailed financial accounting systems. Development aid from development banks and international donor organizations comes with far more strings attached than security funds. Foundation funds, as discussed above, although historically among the most flexible, have gradually come more into line with those of the largest donors. Individual private donations to new, web-savvy organizations may be among the more flexible sources of funds, but they are, to date, relatively small.

Most of the funds for meeting global goals will continue to come from Third World governments, many of which are still working to establish effective and equitable systems for taxing their citizens. More funding for the next generation of schools is expected to come from tax revenues collected from the cohort of children now in primary school. This constitutes a powerful argument for two-track funding today. If no stopgap measures are put in place soon, many of this cohort will graduate illiterate, and their chances of finding jobs and earning income sufficient to raise their families above the poverty line and become taxpayers 15 to 20 years from now will be much reduced.

A FUTURE FOR GLOBAL EDUCATION GOALS?

In 2015 the global community will ratify a new—or not so new—set of global development goals. I am able to predict this with some confidence because the notion of global goals has become so institutionalized that even I, an institutional scholar fully conscious of the socially constructed nature and weaknesses of those goals, find it hard to imagine the international development community without them.

Education will be featured in post-2015 global goals. In 2012 some remarks at high-level international meetings on post-2015 global goals suggested that education might not need to be included in those goals, given that many countries had met the education MDGs (Burnett, 2012). For many in the global education community, particularly those who had been scandalized by the low bar set by the education MDGs, this was a call to arms. In response, education experts began to meet to identify research that might strengthen the case for education and develop prototype goals. Support for individual education as a foundation for all other socioeconomic development runs strongly through other sectors, and education advocates will find much support for retaining education in the post-2015 goals outside the education sector.

The post-2015 global education goals are likely to be stated in comprehensive, aspirational terms. The evidence for selective primary education interventions remains sufficiently ambiguous that defenders of the comprehensive approach can continue to argue that the selectivists have failed to prove their case. As former UNICEF director James P. Grant said it would, the Growth Monitoring-Oral Rehydration-Breast Feeding-Immunization components of the Child Survival initiative indeed served as the catalyst for more global health initiatives in malaria, HIV/AIDS, guinea worm/river blindness, tuberculosis, and other diseases, some of them quite successful. And beyond the health sector, Child Survival, not Health for All, was the catalyst for a global initiative in education.[2] However, Primary School Student Survival does not make most education advocates' hearts beat faster, and the number of international agreements committing countries to provide a more comprehensive approach to education has only increased.

Comprehensive, aspirational goals or not, funding shortages will likely continue to dictate a highly selective de facto program of action. The only Third World country where Health for All or Education for All has been comprehensively achieved since 1980 is perhaps Cuba (Carnoy, 2007). Cuba's achievement was supported with unprecedented amounts of aid per capita from the Soviet Union by an authoritarian government. If indeed there are no other country examples, the best that can be said for the ultimate feasibility and success of the comprehensive approach is that it remains untested. With respect to international development organizations, the evidence to date suggests that they have struggled mightily to support selective approaches and that there is no evidence that any of them alone or together could support a comprehensive one. Those organizations engaged in primary education, moreover, have not identified game-changing innovations and approaches and therefore have no basis on which to estimate the cost of achieving even a selective approach.

Cross-nationally comparable numeric targets for learning indicators will be associated with the selective approach. The Center for Universal Education and its Learning Metrics Task Force attempted between 2011 and 2013 to engage more educators in more venues in virtual consultations in order not to leave the metrics decisions in the hands of the economists. For thoughtful professionals, the decision to accede to the international development field's insatiable hunger for targets is a fraught one. Without estimates of how far and how fast certain levels of funding can advance education for all, securing significant funding for good programs will be difficult. At the same time, experience shows that there is no quantitative target that cannot be weaponized—transformed into a blunt instrument and used to beat teachers and low-level education administrators to achieve it. Such targets have little to do with learning and everything to do with a numbers game being played at the national and international level. Professionals disposed to take their chances with targets, therefore, should strive to ensure that the ones selected are those that appear least likely to distort activities at the grass roots and for which effective strategies to control their misuse are at hand.

In 1968, Albert Hirschman wrote an essay on, among other things, "obstacles to the perception of change" (Hirschman, 1968, p. 926). One of the chief obstacles he discerned was the tendency to treat anything less than full achievement of ambitious goals as a complete failure, possibly an early formulation of his *fracaso*-mania or "failure-mania" thesis. I confess that a decade ago, looking at meager progress toward EFA, the working title of this book was "EFA: Why Isn't It Dead Yet?" Since that time, however, significant progress has been made toward the Dakar Goals for a full primary education for all children by 2015. The notion of measuring learning outcomes, particularly literacy and soon, it is to be hoped, numeracy and essential learning skills, has also advanced. Indeed, the international development field has moved global goals farther and faster than any rational-technical or critical analysis gave us reason to expect. Nor did this progress result simply from one success being built upon another. Rather, in keeping with Hirschman's First Law of the Conservation of Social Energy, many of the projects that succeeded were the work of people previously involved in more ambitious collective undertakings that failed.

Indeed, international development organizations deserve considerable credit for shifting upward the trajectory of the spread of human rights and physical well-being from the one projected by demographers in the early 1970s for many former colonies. Few suggest that the world would have been better off without global development initiatives like Health for All and Education for All. More charge that these organizations could have done far more, better, and faster, but that remains to be proven.

Following a talk on early reading at a large international development organization, a midlevel project officer approached me with great excitement. "I loved your presentation. Next week I'm flying to Country X to negotiate a new early reading program and I need a list of the best reading interventions so I can be sure we put them in the strategy. Where can I find that list?" For a few seconds I fumbled, taken aback by my failure to convey the most fundamental notions about context and innovation. What could I say to this person who was unaware of his bureaucratic baggage and in search of a blueprint? Suddenly I saw bathwater and multiple babies flying through the air in Country X. Then I took a deep breath and invited him to sit down. "What can you tell me," I asked, "about the organizations in Country X?"

Notes

Chapter 1

1. For a thorough description of the use of models, scripts, and identities in neo-institutionalist analysis, see Ramirez (2012). This book refers sparingly to models of mass primary education and of development. Ramirez and I (Chabbott & Ramirez, 2000) first used the term *blueprints* for models for which step-by-step implementation processes had become widely available, such as the international development conferences that produce global goals.

2. See, e.g., Adams & Chen (1981); Bishop (1986); Cummings (1986b); Havelock & Huberman (1978); Lewin & Stuart (1991); Lynch, Modgil, & Modgil (1997); Organisation for Economic Co-operation and Development (OECD), Centre for Educational Research and Innovation (1973); Stromquist & Basile (1999).

3. Francisco O. Ramirez provided the chicken soup analogy (personal communication, October 17, 2013).

4. The nonbinding Declaration of Universal Human Rights was adopted in 1948 and transferred into two binding covenants that most countries ratified in the late 1960s and early 1970s. For copies of these and other human rights treaties and a history of ratifications and accession, see the online UN Treaty Collection at treaties.un.org.

5. The classic definition of the scientific method includes formulating an explicit hypothesis, seeking out measurable evidence, and designing and carrying out experiments that use the evidence to test the hypothesis. This definition is generally less problematic in the natural sciences than in the social sciences. Popper argued that experiments could only approach the truth by eliminating what was false (falsification), rather than proving what was true. For a more complete discussion of Popper and the use of the scientific method in the social sciences, see Tudor (2007).

6. "An idealized market situation in which all information is known to all market participants, and both buyers and sellers are so numerous that each is a price-taker, able to buy or sell any desired quantity without affecting the market price." "Perfect competition" in Black, Hashimzade, and Myles (2009).

7. To which U.S. National Security Advisor Henry Kissinger responded, "But not necessarily our basket case." Transcript of the U.S. Government Interdepartmental Washington Special Actions Group, December 6, 1971. Quoted in Mohammad Rezaul Bari (2008). The etymology of *basket case* is ambiguous; some sources refer to a method of immobilizing mental patients prior to the invention of straitjackets, others as a means of transporting quadriplegics.

8. Probability of dying between birth and exact age 5, expressed as average annual deaths per 1,000 births. See esa.un.org/unpd/wpp/Excel-Data/mortality.htm

9. See "Falsification" in the Blackwood Encyclopedia of Sociology: www .sociologyencyclopedia.com/public/tocnode?query=falsification&widen=1&result _number=1&from=search&fuzzy=0&type=std&id=g9781405124331_yr2012_ chunk_g978140512433112_ss1-7&slop=1

10. See research.brac.net/publications.php

Chapter 2

1. As of mid-2011, the CPR Covenant had not been ratified by China, Nauru, Comoros, Cuba, or São Tome and Principe.

2. As of mid-2011, the United States, South Africa, Belize, Comoros, Cuba, and São Tome and Principe had not ratified the ESCR Covenant.

3. treaties.un.org/Pages/ShowMTDSGDetails.aspx?src=UNTSONLINE&tabid =2&mtdsg_no=IV-3&chapter=4&lang=en#EndDec

4. For a history of UNICEF's Cold War origins and its relationship with the United States, see Black (1996), Jones (2005), and Stein (2007).

5. According to a member of the staff who worked on the meetings, the NGOs appreciated the irony that they, most attached to organizations with strong religious roots, were helping to organize a conference in a Soviet republic where independent religious or even secular civic organizations were not allowed to form (Personal communication, Sheila Tacon Barry, HFA NGO Committee participant, October 1, 2012).

6. "3. includes at least: education concerning prevailing health problems and the methods of preventing and controlling them; promotion of food supply and proper nutrition; an adequate supply of safe water and basic sanitation; maternal and child health care, including family planning; immunization against the major infectious diseases; prevention and control of locally endemic diseases; appropriate treatment of common diseases and injuries; and provision of essential drugs." Article 3, *Declaration of Alma-Ata*.

7. The United Kingdom and the United States withdrew from UNESCO in 1984. The United Kingdom returned in 1997; the United States returned in 2002, but withdrew again in 2011.

8. For example, the Latin American Educational Documentation Network (f. 1972, REDUC) and the (Northern) Research Review and Advisory Group (f. 1977).

9. *The Experiences and Experiments in Education* (1974–1980) was succeeded by the International Bureau of Education's *Educational Innovations and Information* (1980–2006) and by at least two international studies of innovation in education (Adams & Chen, 1981; Havelock & Huberman, 1978).

10. As of this writing, health care in the United States remains largely private and highly fragmented.

11. Other interventions added later—food supplementation (enriched flour, iodized salt, Vitamin A), female education, and family planning—expanded the acronym to GOBI-FFF.

12. The third killer, respiratory infections, was left off the list because UNICEF did not want to encourage the use of antibiotics by informal health providers.

13. WHO's *World Health Report 2008* (2008b) estimated that less than 20% of births and deaths in Africa and Asia were officially registered; 25 years earlier, vital statistics were even less complete.

14. Chapter 6 includes more details on USAID's work with ORT.

Chapter 3

An earlier version of this chapter was published as Chabbott (2007) and benefited greatly from editing by David Post.

1. The way of contrasting the MDGs was originally suggested by John W. Meyer, professor emeritus, Stanford University.

2. For example, Bangladesh met the mid-decade MDGs for education, but in a 2001 assessment of Class V in rural government schools, less than 2% of students achieved minimum levels of the terminal competencies for primary school (Chowdhury, Nath, Choudhury, & Ahmed, 2002).

3. See the OECD's Center for Education Research and Innovation's Brain and Learning Group at www.oecd.org/edu/ceri/centreforeducationalresearchandinnovationceri-brainandlearning.html. In addition, some videotape studies are approaching high levels of precision within classroom studies; see, for example, Stigler (1999).

4. . . . to the perpetual frustration of educators. See Moats (1999).

5. See www.campbellcollaboration.org

6. See www.cochrane.org

7. "Experimental research designs require that all cases are *randomly* allocated to either the experimental group which receives the treatment being tested, or to a *control* group which receives no treatment or an ineffective placebo treatment and hence provides baseline information on spontaneous developments against which the effects of the experimental treatment can be measured" (Marshall, 1994, p. 91, emphasis added).

8. See www.campbellcollaboration.org/lib/index.php?basic_search=1&go= browse_small&search_data%5B0%5D%5Bquery%5D=education&search_data% 5B0%5D%5Bcriteria%5D=title. Not included in this number is an approved protocol for "Parental, Familial, and Community Support Interventions to Improve Children's Literacy in Developing Countries: A Systematic Review."

9. See www.ed.gov/about/offices/list/ies/index.html

10. See ies.ed.gov/ncee/wwc/FindWhatWorks.aspx. NB: This URL opens a search page. Select: Literacy/reading comprehension/PK-G5/Positive or potentially positive/ medium to large scale. The exact number of studies will change as the Clearinghouse updates its data.

11. See search.oecd.org/officialdocuments/publicdisplaydocumentpdf/?cote= EDU/CERI/CD/RD%282004%291&docLanguage=En

12. For more information on other research using RCTs to analyze education interventions in Colombia, India, Kenya, and Egypt, see http://www .povertyactionlab.org/search/apachesolr_search?filters=type%3Aevaluation%20

sm_cck_field_themes%3A2. For more on randomized field trials in general, see National Research Council (2004).

13. A few exceptions, however, come to mind, including the Khan Academy and Kumon tutoring centers.

14. Thanks to Richard A. Cash, William B. and Quaneta Greenough III, W. Henry and "Bunny" Mosley, David R. Nalin, David Sachar, David and Jean Sack, and Josephine and R. Bradley Sack for special help with this section.

15. Medicine distinguishes between watery diarrhea and more solid dysentery.

16. Some earlier partly effective treatments could cure up to 70% of the cases. David Nalin, personal communication, June 28, 2005.

17. SEATO members included Australia, France, New Zealand, Pakistan (including East Pakistan, now Bangladesh), the Philippines, Thailand, the United Kingdom, and the United States.

18. www.rehydrate.org

19. Chapter 6 addresses this diffusion process.

Chapter 4

1. Bangladesh had the last recorded case of smallpox *major* in the world in 1975. See www.ncbi.nlm.nih.gov/pubmed/22188934

2. This section is broadly informed by several first-person accounts: Chen (1983); F. H. Abed in Smillie (2009); Rohde, J. (2005c); Rohde, C. (2014).

3. Since 1977, BRAC's Research and Evaluation Division (RED) has published hundreds of internal studies. Many are available at research.brac.net/publications. php

4. BRAC health programs focused on 1) diarrhea/cholera, 2) dysentery-amoebic, bacillary, 3) worms, 4) typhoid and paratyphoid, 5) ulcer, 6) tetanus, 7) pneumonia, 8) leprosy, 9) tuberculosis, 10) scabies, 11) malaria, 12) measles, 13) smallpox and chickenpox. This includes the 10 illnesses that WHO had identified as manageable by community level health workers, plus three others prevalent in Bangladesh (Zaman & Karim, 2005, p. 37).

5. See en.wikipedia.org/wiki/Barefoot_doctor

6. In the 1980s, as the government geared up its family planning program, BRAC scaled back to cover only its village organization members, making referrals to government family planning clinics as those became established near villages with BRAC groups.

7. Two community-based health care innovations in Bangladesh were featured in one of the volumes of case studies prepared for the Health for All conference (Djukonovic & Mach, 1975), but it appears that both were designed and implemented by NGOs.

8. Much of the material in this section is drawn from Chowdhury and Cash (1996).

9. In many parts of the world, without a well-established system of law and order, particularly following large-scale conflicts such as the Bangladesh War of Independence, bandits, predatory elites, and uncontrolled gangs of young men are

common hazards in rural areas. In these settings, the distance that children, particularly girls from poor families, can safely travel to school may be severely circumscribed. For examples in Bangladesh in the first decade of independence, see Hartmann and Boyce (1985).

10. Since the areas most in need had few structures, roads, or public transportation, BRAC staff camped out nearby.

11. All statistics collected during Bangladesh's 1st decade were affected by the successive catastrophes that marred the nation's venture into independence; thus, all statistics should be treated as estimates.

12. All approximations from World Bank sources: Primary Education Project (PEP I, 1980–1985, US$40 million; PEP II, 1985–1990, US$100 million); General Education Project (GEP, 1991–1997, US$159 million), Primary Education Development Project (PEDP I, 1998–2003, US$ 741 million; PEDP II, 2004–2009, US$650 million). The government began disbursing its principal commodity (food) and later its cash transfer program for the poor through Food for Education and later Primary School Stipend programs.

13. These children are the first in their families to attend primary school.

14. The following account draws largely on first-person interviews in 2006, 2007, and 2012 with staff who were most active in the establishment of the dominant model that emerged from this experimentation: BRAC's Nonformal Primary Education (NFPE) program.

15. After independence, the spelling of Dacca was changed to Dhaka.

16. The Indian Institute of Education (f. 1948) was founded by J. P. Naik (1907–1981), who was also founding member-secretary of the Indian Council for Social Science Research (ICSSR); chief author of UNESCO's Karachi Plan (1959) and Addis Ababa Plan (1961) of universal primary education; and author of the report "Health for All by the Year 2000," under the aegis of the ICSSR and the Indian Council for Medical Research. See www.iiepune.org/html/vision.htm

17. Several multigrade school models in India (RIVER) and Latin America (*Escuela Nueva*) use cards for programmed learning, allowing children to proceed through the curriculum at their own pace, without textbooks. Where such programs serve largely illiterate communities, parents sometimes request some books that the children can carry back and forth to school. The institution of the textbook is a strong one.

18. Meaning "Let's read."

19. The name of these types of schools changed over time: Kishor Kishoree (KK or adolescent boys and girls) classes, Basic Education for Older Children (BEOC), and BRAC Adolescent Primary Schools (BAPS).

20. See Note 9.

Chapter 5

1. See, for example, the Institute for International Education Planning's series on capacity development strategies, including one report on Bangladesh, Riddell (2011).

2. Political science has a large literature on decentralization and accountability relevant to democratization and neoliberalism; this analysis focuses exclusively on the management and sociology of organizations literature.

3. As discussed in Chapter 4, this tendency is what Hirschman (1975) calls failure-mania. The tongue-in-cheek "Steps in the life of a project," widely circulated in the international development field, reflects a similar perspective: 1. Wild enthusiasm; 2. Disillusionment; 3. Confusion; 4. Panic; 5. Search for the guilty; 6. Punishment of the innocent; 7. Promotion of nonparticipants.

4. BRAC was likely one of the cases that Korten and Jain had in mind when they proposed this typology for NGOs working in Third World development. See, for example, Jain (1997), which showcases NFPE and another alternative primary education program implemented by another Bangladeshi NGO, Gonoshahajjo Sangstha (GSS).

5. This section draws largely on Chowdhury and Cash (1996), supplemented by reports, working papers, monographs, and publications by BRAC and other researchers, many of which may be found at research.brac.net/#.

6. In Bangladesh these schools include allopathy (modern Western), homeopathy, ayurvedic, unani, and folk.

7. The first 3-year NFPE effort following the pilot was simply called "NFPE." The word "project" is added here to distinguish it from the three phases of NFPE scale-up that followed.

8. See, for example, S. Chowdhury et al. (1988).

9. See, for example, Khan and Chowdhury (1991, 1993).

10. In the late 1980s, donors to BRAC's rural development program agreed to join a consortium that would accept one set of progress reports, audits, evaluations, and proposals.

11. Teacher training for one cycle during Phase 1 scale-up totaled about 56 days, including:

Preservice	12 residential
Orientation before Grade 1	3 inservice
Refreshers, end of Months 1 and 2	4 inservice
Refresher, end of Year 1	4 inservice
Refresher, end of Year 2	3 inservice
Refreshers, monthly when no other training	~30 inservice

In addition, POs visited first-cycle schools twice weekly and at least weekly for subsequent cycles, totaling 134–268 supervisory visits over 3 years (BRAC NFPE, 1997, pp. 14, 19).

12. See www.campebd.org

13. For a side-by-side table comparing key features of government and NFPE schools in 2007, see Ahmed, Ahmed, Ahmed, and Ahmed, (2007, p. 97). This table shows NFPE with five grades, but at the time of the *Together for Education* proposal, NFPE covered only three grades.

14. Between 1990 and 1995, physical facilities including furniture and fixtures constituted 88–92% of development expenditure for primary education (Ahmad, 1997).

15. In 1995 teacher and staff compensation constituted 95.7% of revenue (domestic) expenditure on primary education (Ahmed, 1997).

16. For a contemporaneous case study of the effects of bureaucracy at all levels of the formal primary education system, see Hossain (1994). Other, more recent studies at the school level had similar findings (Tietjen, Rahman, & Spaulding, 2004).

17. See "Efficient and Cost-Effective" subsection below for more on comparative quality of learning.

18. See Chapter 2 in this volume.

19. As was expected, NFPE students performed much better in life skills, and students of other schools performed somewhat better in mental arithmetic and writing (Chowdhury, Mohsin, & Nath, 1992).

20. From 1993 to 2000, BRAC research reports on education averaged 10 reports per year, peaking at 19 studies in 1999. See www.bracresearch.org/publications.php for a complete, searchable list of many of BRAC's Research and Evaluation Division studies.

21. Surveyors failed to keep the survey sites anonymous. The NFPE director feared that publicizing the relatively poor performance of government schools might have had negative repercussions for those schools that had cooperated with the survey, and, by extension, the nearby NFPE schools. The complete Rahman Rahman Huq (1992) report was not publicly released.

22. Later, in 2002, the Primary and Mass Education Division became the Ministry of Primary and Mass Education.

23. Policymakers may have an aversion to education research they themselves have not commissioned. For the Bangladesh case, see Unterhalter, Ross, and Alam (2003).

24. For an early history and review of the IMPACT project in Bangladesh, see Cummings (1986a).

25. A 2004 report found that errors of inclusion and exclusion were large, and a large proportion of nonpoor households met the official stipend targeting criteria (Ahmed & Taniya, 2004).

26. At first, students were encouraged to read the books at home, and the subject was not taught during school hours until later, when the NFPE curriculum aligned more closely to the formal curriculum. Foreign donors were unwilling to fund the religion curriculum in NFPE.

27. We use here the same categories of scaling up as for *lobon-gur*, but, for the sake of chronology, in a different order.

28. Originally intended to fund more schools.

29. As described earlier, in 1990, 16 NGOs—accounting for 90% of the nonformal education funding in the Bangladesh—formed the Campaign for Mass and Primary Education (CAMPE, f. 1990), with BRAC's director as its first chairman.

30. A sample of NGO schools, including a few from NFPE, constituted one comparison group. BRAC researchers later tested an oversample of NFPE schools comparable to the subgroup "formal schools in rural areas," the latter was reported on in tables in the *Education Watch* annexes (Ahmad & Haque, 2011; Nath, 2000, 2006).

31. By monitoring leading indicators of disease at regular intervals at key locations, health planners try to get a head start on epidemics or quickly identify breaks in vaccine coverage.

32. The basic education criterion consisted of correct responses to three of four oral reading comprehension questions, three of four mental arithmetic problems, and seven of ten life skills questions, and conveying a simple message in writing (Chowdhury, Zieghan, Haque, Shrestha, & Ahmed, 1994).

33. Of the 53 competencies in the formal curriculum in 2001, 26 could be measured by a paper-and-pencil test.

34. Indeed, a Bangladeshi sociologist comparing NFPE and formal classrooms in rural areas declared NFPE's "Montessori-like" (Khan & Arefeen, 1992). Western politicians, including Tony Blair and Bill Clinton, expressed delight with NFPE classrooms.

35. Most secondary schools, encompassing Grades 6 and above, are privately owned and operated in Bangladesh.

36. Traditionally, poor families might scrape together funds sufficient to send one or two boys to formal school, but few such families sent all children.

37. In real 2009 dollars, the combined value of NFPE pilot—NFPE 3, with the addition of Grades 4 and 5 to most schools and dozens of other new activities, was about $303 million. Source: author calculation, Table 5.2.

38. The availability of stipends at the secondary level appears to have increased Bangladeshi parents' motivation to support their girls through primary school. See Tables 5.1 and 5. 2.

Chapter 6

1. Packets often included step-by-step instructions in pictures, so that the ability to read text was not required.

2. Bicarbonate was part of the WHO-approved formula. Effective ORS can be made without it.

3. The acronym for the core activities of the Child Survival initiative: Growth monitoring, Oral rehydration, Breast feeding, and Immunization.

4. Much of this section was previously published in Chabbott (2008).

5. Intergovernmental organization.

6. Later many staff from Lok Jombish, an Indian rural development NGO with a well-known community school model included in the Oxfam-supported Varma and Malviya study, would visit BRAC often. I have found no evidence, however, that the BRAC Education Program was involved in these visits.

7. Official exchange rate (2005): 64.328 Taka = US$1

8. In April 2005, three Afghan women associated with BRAC were stoned to death in Baghlan, and in January 2006 an Afghan engineer working for BRAC was also killed. As a result, in July 2006 BRAC withdrew from southern Afghanistan.

9. "Interagency" in the title was later changed to "International."

Chapter 7

1. Formerly the Operations Evaluation Department of the World Bank.

2. Hence the name of a similar U.S. policy, "No Child Left Behind," which has not achieved this goal.

3. RTI International is a large, interdisciplinary, nonprofit organization best known in the education sector of the international development field for its quantitative analysis.

4. "The amount of practice required to activate the automatic pathway depends on the consistency between letters and sounds. . . . Languages that involve complex spelling rules require more proactive instruction for automaticity and also faster reading for timely comprehension. . . . Overall, English-medium students require 2.5 or more years of literacy learning to master the recognition of familiar words and simple decoding that is learned in one year for languages with simpler spelling rules [e.g., Italian]" (Abadzi, 2006, p. 30).

5. http://www.youtube.com/watch?v=-BxL1aqb6mY , accessed 5/21/2014.

6. In the early years of the community, most understood prereading foundations as phonological awareness, print awareness, alphabet knowledge, and oral language. Reading foundations included phonemic awareness, phonics, fluency, vocabulary, and comprehension. Later, Abadzi, citing Share (2008), argued that phonemic awareness and oral comprehension were relevant for English, but not for many other languages, and that phonological awareness is more correlational than causal. She proposed to reformulate the foundational components to letters, running text, and comprehension.

7. Languages vary in the number and size of discrete chunks of text and patterns of sounds that learners must recognize before they can read fluently (Ziegler & Goswami, 2005). Reading fluently is a necessary but not sufficient precursor to the ultimate goal of reading instruction: reading with comprehension.

8. The Project on Universal Basic and Secondary Education (2001–2006, UBASE) at the American Academy of Arts and Sciences in Boston, Mass., and the Center for Universal Education (2002–, CUE) now at the Brookings Institution in Washington, D.C.

9. The goal of the EDDATA project was to improve "the accuracy, timeliness, and accessibility, [and use] of data for basic education policy and program planning" for USAID headquarters as well as its missions and governments anywhere in the global South.

10. The name "Test of Oral Reading Fluency" is copyrighted by a U.S. organization.

11. See timssandpirls.bc.edu/pirls2011/international-results-pirls.html

12. Several readers of this manuscript tried to make the case here that the process for establishing standards for oral reading fluency and comprehension by language are more subjective than for anthropometry for children by ethnic group. The issue is beyond my expertise in both subjects, but I think I can say that most educators would be shocked by how much margin for error remains in anthropometry.

13. For example, see Jessee et al. (2003), Miske (2003), Johnson, Hayter, and Broadfoot (2000), and Williams (1998).

14. See www.molteno.co.za/about-molteno/about-us.

15. See www.prathamusa.org/about-us/history.

16. Save the Children-U.S. is one of 30 Save the Children member organizations that since 2010 operate as one entity in Third World countries: Save the Children International.

17. Like RTI's EDDATA program, in some countries, such as the Philippines, Save's *Literacy Boost* carries out reading assessments but supports no special reading interventions.

18. See plan-international.org/what-we-do/education.

19. See www.cal.org/topics/id/.

20. Major donors to education created the Fast Track Initiative in 2002 to consolidate and streamline funding to support credible strategies for achieving the education MDG proposed by countries facing substantial performance and funding gaps. FTI was later rebranded as the Global Partnership for Education.

21. See, e.g., El Centro de Investigación y Acción Educativa Social (CIASES) in Managua, Nicaragua.

22. See www.urc-chs.com/news?newsItemID=390#sthash.IPS8aVSE.dpuf

23. I.e., students and schools that are available within the researchers' time frame, not randomized.

Chapter 8

1. See www.urc-chs.com/news?newsItemID=390#sthash.IPS8aVSE.dpuf.

2. See Chapter 2.

References

Abadzi, H. (2003). *Improving adult literacy outcomes: Lessons from cognitive research for developing countries* (Directions in Development). Washington, DC: World Bank.

Abadzi, H. (2006). *Efficient learning for the poor: Insights from the frontier of cognitive neuroscience* (Operations Evaluation Division). Washington, DC: World Bank.

Abadzi, H. (2007). *Absenteeism and beyond: Instructional time loss and consequences* (Operations Evaluation Division). Washington, DC: World Bank.

Abadzi, H. (2008). Efficient learning for the poor: New insights into literacy acquisition for children. *International Review of Education, 54*(5-6), 581–604.

Abadzi, H. (2012). *Developing cross-language metrics for reading fluency measurement: Some issues and options.* Washington, DC: EFA Fast Track Initiative.

Abadzi, H. (2013). Education for all in low-income countries: A crucial role for cognitive scientists. *British Journal of Education, Society & Behavioural Science, 3*(4), 1–23.

Abadzi, H. (2014). How to improve schooling outcomes in low-income countries? The challenges and hopes of cognitive neuroscience. *Peabody Journal of Education, 89*(1), 58–69.

Abadzi, H., Crouch, L., Echegaray, M., Pasco, C., & Sampe, J. (2005). Monitoring basic skills acquisition through rapid learning assessments: A case study from Peru. *Prospects, XXXV*(2), 138–159.

Abbott, A. (1988). *The system of professions: An essay on the division of expert labor.* Chicago, IL: University of Chicago Press.

Adams, R. S., & Chen, D. (1981). *The process of educational innovation: An international perspective.* Paris: Kogan Page/UNESCO.

Adamson, P. (2001). The mad American. In R. Jolly (Ed.), *Jim Grant: UNICEF visionary* (pp. 19–36). Florence, Italy: UNICEF Innocenti Research Centre.

Ahmad, A., & Haque, I. (2010). *Economic and social analysis of primary education in Bangladesh: A study of BRAC interventions and mainstream schools.* Dhaka, Bangladesh: BRAC.

Ahmad, A., & Haque, I. (2011). *Economic and social analysis of primary education in Bangladesh: A study of BRAC interventions and mainstream schools.* Dhaka: BRAC Research and Evaluation Division.

Ahmed, A. U., & Taniya, S. (2004). *Assessing the performance of conditional cash transfer programs for girls and boys in primary and secondary schools in*

Bangladesh (Partnership for Sustainable Strategies on Girls' Education). Washington, DC: International Institute for Food Policy Research.

Ahmed, M. (1997). Financing of primary education. In A. K. Jalaluddin & A. M. R. Chowdhury (Eds.), *Getting started: Universalising quality primary education in Bangladesh* (pp. 148–167). Dhaka, Bangladesh: University Press Limited.

Ahmed, M. (1980). BRAC: Building human infrastructures to serve the rural poor. In P. H. Coombs (Ed.), *Meeting the needs of the rural poor: The integrated community-based approach* (pp. 362–469). New York, NY: Pergamon & International Council for Educational Development.

Ahmed, M. (1984). The education revolution in Tanzania. *Assignment Children: Going to Scale for Child Survival and Development, 65/68*, 225–245.

Ahmed, M., Ahmed, K. S., Ahmed, N. I., & Ahmed, R. (2007). *Access to education in Bangladesh: Country analytic review of primary and secondary education* (Consortium for Research on Educational Access, Transitions and Equity). Sussex, UK: University of Sussex, and Dhaka, Bangladesh: BRAC University, Institute of Educational Development.

Ahmed, M., Chabbott, C., Joshi, A., & Pande, R. (1993). *Primary education for all: Learning from the BRAC experience*. Washington, DC: Academy for Educational Development.

Ahmed, M., & Coombs, P. H. (Eds.). (1975). *Education for rural development: Case studies for planners*. New York: Praeger.

Ali, S. (1948). *Deshi, Bideshi [Of this country, Not of this country]* (In Bangla). Dhaka, Bangladesh: Unknown.

Al-Samarrai, S., Bennell, P., & Colclough, C. (2002). *From projects to SWAps: An evaluation of British aid to primary education, 1998–2001*. London: Department of International Development.

Alam, M., Begum, K., & Raihan, A. (1997). Efficiency of primary education in Bangladesh. In A. K. Jalaluddin & A. M. R. Chowdhury (Eds.), *Getting started: Universalising quality primary education in Bangladesh*. Dhaka, Bangladesh: University Press Limited.

Anderson, M. B. (1992). *Education for All: What are we waiting for?* New York, NY: UNICEF.

Argyris, C., & Schön, D. A. (1978). *Organizational learning: A theory of action perspective*. Reading, MA: Addison-Wesley.

Asian Development Bank. (2007). *Bangladesh: Country operations business plan (2008–2010)*. Manila, Philippines: Asian Development Bank.

Aziz, K. M. A., & Mosley, W. H. (1994). Historical perspective and methodology of the Matlab project. In V. Fauveau (Ed.), *Matlab: Women, children and health* (pp. 29–50). Dhaka, Bangladesh: Pioneer Printing.

Banerjee, A., Banerji, R., Duflo, E., Glennerster, R., Kenniston, D., Khemani, S., et al. (2007). Can information campaigns raise awareness and local participation in primary education? *Economic and Political Weekly, 42*(15), 1365–1372.

Banerjee, A. V., Banerji, R., Duflo, E., Glennerster, R., & Khemani, S. (2008). *Pitfalls of participatory programs: Evidence from a randomized evaluation in education in India*. Washington, DC: World Bank.

Banerjee, A., Cole, S., Duflo, E., & Linden, L. (2003). *Remedying education: Evidence from two randomized experiences in India* (Poverty Action Lab Paper No. 4). Cambridge, MA: Poverty Action Lab.

Bangladesh Forum for Educational Development. (1992). *Findings of the evaluation study on the Facilitation and Assistance Programme on Education (FAPE) of BRAC: A brief* [Manuscript]. Dhaka, Bangladesh: UNICEF.

Bari, M. R. (2008, October 29). The basket case. *The Daily Star* [Dhaka, Bangladesh], p. 1.

Barua, D. (2003a, September-December). Dr. Dhiman Barua receives lifetime achievement award. *Glimpse, 2*.

Barua, D. (2003b). Speech to ASCODD upon receipt of lifetime achievement award (excerpt). In J. Sack & M. Rahim (Eds.), *Smriti: ICDDR,B in Memory* (pp. 137–138). Dhaka, Bangladesh: International Center for Diarrheal Disease Research/Bangladesh.

Barua, D. (2009). Miracle cure for an old scourge. *Bulletin of the World Health Organization, 87*, 81–82.

Baulch, B. (2011). The medium-term impact of the primary education stipend in Bangladesh. *Journal of Development Effectiveness, 3*(2), 243–262.

Begum, K., Akhter, S., & Rahman, S. (1988). *An evaluation of BRAC's primary education program* [draft mimeo]. Dhaka, Bangladesh: World Bank.

Behar, R. (2012, July 16). World Bank mired in dysfunction: Mess awaits new head. *Forbes, 4*.

Bell, D. (1987). Child survival: The Role of UNICEF. In R. Cash, G. Keusch, & J. Lamstain (Eds.), *Child health and survival: The UNICEF GOBI-FFF program* (pp. 251–253). Beckenham, England: Croom Helm.

Berger, P. L. (1999). The desecularization of the world: A global overview. In P. L. Berger (Ed.), *The desecularization of the world: Resurgent religion and world politics* (pp. 1–18). Washington, DC: Ethics & Public Policy Center and Wm. B. Eerdmans.

Berger, P. L., Berger, B., & Kellner, H. (1973). *The homeless mind: Modernization and consciousness*. New York, NY: Vintage.

Berger, P. L., & Luckmann, T. (1967). *The social construction of reality: A treatise in the sociology of knowledge*. New York, NY: Anchor Books (Doubleday).

Berman, P. A. (1982). Selective primary health care: Is efficient sufficient? *Social Science and Medicine, 16*, 1054–1059.

Bhatia, S., Cash, R. A., & Cornaz, I. (1983). *Evaluation of the Oral Therapy Education Programme of the Bangladesh Rural Advancement Committee*. Berne, Switzerland: Swiss Development Cooperation.

Bill and Melinda Gates Foundation. (2006). *Improving the quality of learning outcomes in the developing world* (Request for Proposals). Seattle, WA: Author.

Bishop, G. (1986). *Innovation in education*. London, England: Macmillan.

Black, J., Hashimzade, N., & Myles, G. (2009). *A dictionary of economics*. Available at www.oxfordreference.com/views/ENTRY.html?subview=Main&entry=t19.e2315

Black, M. (1996). *Children first: The story of UNICEF, past and present*. Oxford, England: Oxford University and UNICEF.

Boeren, A., Latif, A. H., & Stromquist, N. (1995). *Evaluation of the expansion of BRAC's Non-Formal Primary Education program, Phase I (1993–95)* [final mimeo]. Dhaka, Bangladesh: BRAC Donor Liaison Office.

BRAC. (2006). *BRAC 2005* (Annual Report). Dhaka, Bangladesh: Author.

BRAC Education Programme. (2002). *Technical assistance outside Bangladesh for replicating NFPE* (BEP progress report). Dhaka, Bangladesh: Author.

BRAC Non-Formal Primary Education Programme. (1997). *[Final] Report to donors on Phase 1 (January 1993–March 1996)*. Dhaka, Bangladesh: BRAC.

BRAC Non-Formal Primary Education Programme. (1999). *[Final] Report to donors on Phase 2 (April 1996–May 1999)*. Dhaka, Bangladesh: BRAC.

Bransford, J. D., Brown, A. L., & Pellegrino, J. W. (Eds.). (2000). *How people learn: Brain, mind, experience, and school* (expanded ed.). Washington, DC: National Academy Press.

Brinkerhoff, D., & Coston, J. (1999). International development management in a globalized world. *Public Administration Review, 59*(4), 343–362.

Brock-Utne, B. (2007). Language of instruction and academic performance: New insights from research in Tanzania and South Africa. *International Review of Education, 53*, 509–530.

Bromley, P. P., & Andina, M. (2009). Standardizing chaos: A neo-institutional analysis of the INEE minimum standards for education in emergencies, chronic crises and early reconstruction. *Compare, 40*(5), 575–588.

Burnett, N. (2012). *Will there be education goals after 2015?* Washington, DC: Results for Development.

Bryant, C., & White, L. G. (1982). *Managing development in the Third World*. Boulder, CO: Westview.

Bryant, J. (1969). *Health and the developing world*. Ithaca, NY: Cornell University.

Bryce, J., Victora, C. G., & Black, R. E. (2013). The unfinished agenda in child survival. *Lancet, 382*(9897), 1049–1059.

Carnoy, M. (1974). *Education as cultural imperialism*. New York, NY: David McKay.

Carnoy, M. (2007). *Cuba's academic advantage: Why students in Cuba do better in school*. Stanford, CA: Stanford University Press.

Cash, R. A. (2003). Putting ORS into the Matlab field station. In J. Sack & M. Rahim (Ed.), *Smriti: ICDDR,B in memory* (pp. 85–86). Dhaka, Bangladesh: ICDDR,B.

Cash, R., Keusch, G., & Lamstain, J. (Eds.). (1987). *Child health and survival: The UNICEF GOBI-FFF program*. Beckenham, England: Croom Helm Ltd.

Centers for Disease Control and Prevention [U.S.]. (1983). International notes diarrheal diseases control program: Global activities, 1981–1982. *Morbidity and Mortality Weekly Report, 32*(25), 330–333.

Chabbott, C. (2003). *Constructing education for development: International organizations and Education for All.* New York, NY: RoutledgeFalmer.

Chabbott, C. (2006). *Accelerating early grades reading in high priority EFA countries: A desk review.* Washington, DC: USAID/American Institutes for Research.

Chabbott, C. (2007). Carrot soup, magic bullets and scientific research for education and development. *Comparative Education Review, 51*(1), 71–94.

Chabbott, C. (2008). BRAC goes global. In L. Chisholm & G. Steiner-Khamsi (Eds.), *South-south: Educational development among equals?* (pp. 192–209). New York, NY: Teachers College Press.

Chabbott, C., & Ramirez, F. (2000). Development and education. In M. T. Hallinan (Ed.), *Handbook of the sociology of education* (pp. 163–187). New York, NY: Kluwer-Plenum.

Chapman, D. W. (2001). *A review of evaluations of UNICEF education activities (1994–2000)* [Internal]. New York, NY: UNICEF.

Chapman, D. W., & Quijada, J. J. (2008). *An analysis of USAID assistance to basic education in the developing world, 1990–2005.* Washington, DC: USAID.

Chatterjee, H. N. (1953). Control of vomiting in cholera and oral replacement fluid. *Lancet, 265*(6795), 1063.

Chen, M. A. (1983). *A quiet revolution: Women in transition in rural Bangladesh.* Cambridge, MA: Schenkman.

Chiappe, P., Siegel, L. S., & Gottardo, A. (2002). Reading related skills of kindergartners from diverse linguistic backgrounds. *Applied Psycholinguistics, 23,* 95–116.

Chiejine, I. (2005, December 30). Taking community schools to children in rural Sierra Leone. Available at www.UNICEF.org/infobycountry/sierraleone_30628.html

Chowdhury, A. M. R. (1992). *Assessment of basic competencies of children in Bangladesh: A status paper* (draft). Dhaka, Bangladesh: UNICEF/Dhaka.

Chowdhury, A. M. R., Alam, M. A., & Ahmed, J. (2006). Development knowledge and experience—from Bangladesh to Afghanistan and beyond. *Bulletin of the World Health Organization, 84*(8), 677–682.

Chowdhury, A. M. R., & Cash, R. A. (1996). *A simple solution: Teaching millions to treat diarrhea at home.* Dhaka, Bangladesh: University Press Limited.

Chowdhury, A. M. R., Choudhury, R. K., & Nath, S. R. (Eds.). (1999). *Hope not complacency: State of primary education in Bangladesh.* Dhaka, Bangladesh: University Press, Limited.

Chowdhury, A. M. R., Choudhury, R. K., Nath, S. R., Ahmed, M., & Alam, M. (Eds.). (2001). *A question of quality: State of primary education in Bangladesh: Major findings: A synthesis* (vol. 1). Dhaka, Bangladesh: University Press Ltd. and Campaign for Popular Education.

Chowdhury, A. M. R., Chowdhury, S., Islam, M., Islam, A., & Vaughan, J. (1997). Control of tuberculosis by community health workers in Bangladesh. *Lancet, 350*(9072), 169–172.

Chowdhury, A. M. R., & Faruk, K. N. (1982). *A survey method for monitoring a behavioural change.* Dhaka, Bangladesh: BRAC Research and Evaluation Division.

Chowdhury, A. M. R., Karim, F., Cash, R., & Bhuiya, A. (1994). *Sustainability of health education: The case of Oral Rehydration Therapy in Bangladesh.* Dhaka, Bangladesh: BRAC.

Chowdhury, A. M. R., Karim, F., Sarkar, S. K., Cash, R. A., Bhuiya, A., et al. (1997). Status of ORT in Bangladesh: How widely is it used? *Health Policy & Planning, 12*(1), 58–66.

Chowdhury, A. M. R., Mohsin, M., & Nath, S. R. (1992). *Assessment of basic education of children in Bangladesh* (draft). Dhaka, Bangladesh: BRAC Research and Evaluation Division.

Chowdhury, A. M. R., & Nath, S. R. (1999). Learning achievement of children. In A. M. R. Chowdhury, R. K. Choudhury, & S. R. Nath (Eds.), *Hope not complacency: State of primary education in Bangladesh* (vol. 1, pp. 35–49). Dhaka, Bangladesh: University Press, Limited.

Chowdhury, A. M. R., Nath, S. R., Choudhury, R. K., & Ahmed, M. (Eds.). (2002). *Renewed hope, daunting challenges: State of primary education in Bangladesh 2001.* Dhaka, Bangladesh: University Press, Limited.

Chowdhury, A. M. R., Zieghan, L., Haque, N., Shrestha, G. L., & Ahmed, Z. (1994). Assessing basic competencies: A practical methodology. *International Review of Education, 40*(6), 437–455.

Chowdhury, F., & Chowdhury, A. (1978). Use patterns of oral contraceptives in rural Bangladesh. *Bangladesh Development Studies, 6*(3), 271–300.

Chowdhury, S., et al. (1988). *Baseline survey in 20 villages in Manikganj prior to opening of non-formal schools.* Dhaka, Bangladesh: BRAC Research and Evaluation Division.

Clemens, M. A. (2004). *The long walk to school: International education goals in historical perspective* (Working Paper No. 37). Washington, DC: Center for Global Development.

Coalition for Evidence-Based Policy. (2003). *Identifying and implementing educational practices supported by rigorous evidence: A user friendly guide.* Washington, DC: National Center for Education Evaluation and Regional Assistance, Institute of Education Science, U.S. Department of Education.

Cole, W. M., & Ramirez, F. O. (2013). Conditional decoupling: Assessing the impact of national human rights institutions, 1981–2004. *American Sociological Review, 20*(10), 1–24.

Communications Initiative. (1999). Interview with Christian Clark [on *Meena*] [Electronic Version]. Available at www.comminit.com/node/149534

Cook, T. D. (2003). Why have education evaluators chosen not to do randomized experiments? *Annals of the American Academy of Political and Social Political Science, 589,* 114–149.

Coombs, P. H. (1968). *The world educational crisis: A systems analysis*. New York, NY: Oxford University Press.

Coombs, P. H. (Ed.). (1980). *Meeting the needs of the rural poor: The integrated community-based approach*. New York: Pergamon & International Council for Educational Development.

Coombs, P. H., & Ahmed, M. (1974a). *Attacking rural poverty: How nonformal education can help*. Baltimore, MD: International Council for Educational Development for the World Bank.

Coombs, P. H., & Ahmed, M. (1974b). *Building new educational strategies to serve rural children and youth*. New York, NY & Essex, CT: UNICEF and the International Council for Educational Development.

Coombs, P. H., Ahmed, M., & Prosser, R. (1973). *New paths to learning for rural children and youth*. New York, NY & Essex, CT: UNICEF and the International Council for Educational Development.

Crouch, L., & Gove, A. (2006). *Concept note: Toward improving global education quality*. Washington, DC: Research Triangle Institute.

Cueto, M. (2004). The origins of primary health care and selective primary health care. *American Journal of Public Health, 94*(11), 1864–1875.

Cummings, W. K. (1986a). Bangladesh's IMPACT. In W. K. Cummings (Ed.), *Low-cost primary education: Implementing innovation in six nations* (pp. 74–79). Ottawa, Canada: International Development Research Centre.

Cummings, W. K. (1986b). *Low-cost primary education: Implementing innovation in six nations*. Ottawa, Canada: International Development Research Centre.

Cummings, W. K., Dall, F., Fiske, E., & Al-Husainy, S. M. (1993). *BRAC appraisal: Feasibility of first [NFPE] expansion phase* [mimeo]. Dhaka, Bangladesh: UNICEF-Dhaka.

Cummins, J. (1979). Linguistic interdependence and the educational development of bilingual children. *Review of Educational Research, 49*, 225–251.

Cutting, W. (1977). Rehydration solutions and domestic measurements. *Lancet, 2*, 663–664.

Davidson, M., & Hobbs, J. (2013). Delivering reading intervention to the poorest children: The case of Liberia and EGRA-plus, a primary grade reading assessment and intervention. *International Journal of Educational Development, 33*(3), 283–294.

Davidson, M., Korda, M., & Collins, O. W. (2011). Teachers' use of EGRA for continuous assessment: The case of EGRA plus: Liberia. In A. Gove & A. Wetterberg (Eds.), *Early grade reading assessment: Applications and interventions to improve basic literacy* (p. 24). Research Triangle Park, NC: Research Triangle Institute.

Delamonica, E., Mehrotra, S., & Vandemoortele, J. (2004). Education for All: How much will it cost? *Development and Change, 35*(1), 3–31.

Delors, J., & The International Commission on Education for the Twenty-First Century. (1996). *Learning: The treasure within* (final). Paris, France: UNESCO.

DiMaggio, P. J. (1988). Interest and agency in institutional theory. In L. Zucker (Ed.), *Institutional patterns and organizations* (pp. 3–21). Cambridge, MA: Ballinger.

DiMaggio, P. J., & Powell, W. W. (1983, April). The iron cage revisited: Institutional isomorphism and collective rationality in organizational fields. *American Sociological Review, 48*, 147–160.

Djukonovic, V., & Mach, E. P. (Eds.). (1975). *Alternative approaches to meeting basic health needs of the populations in developing countries*. Geneva, Switzerland: World Health Organization.

Dove, L. (1981). The political context of education in Bangladesh: 1971–80. In P. Broadfoot, C. Brock, & W. Tulasiewicz (Eds.), *Politics of educational change: An international survey* (pp. 165–182). London, England: Croom Helm.

Drori, G. S., Meyer, J. W., & Hwang, H. (Eds.). (2006). *Globalization and organization: World society and organizational change*. Oxford, England: Oxford University Press.

Ellerbrock, T. (1981). Oral replacement therapy in rural Bangladesh with home ingredients. *Tropical Doctor, 11*, 179–184.

Ellul, J. (1964). *The technological society*. New York, NY: Alfred Knopf. (Original work published 1954)

Farazi, A. H. (1983). *The Oral Therapy Programme: A micro-study of beliefs and practices*. Dhaka, Bangladesh: BRAC Research and Evaluation Division.

Faure, E., & The International Commission on the Development of Education. (1972). *Learning to be* (final). Paris, France: UNESCO.

Feuer, M. J., Towne, L., & Shavelson, R. J. (2002). Scientific culture and educational research. *Educational Researcher, 31*(8), 4–14.

Filmer, D., Hasan, A., & Pritchett, L. (2006). *A millennium development goal: Measuring real progress in education* (Working Paper No. 97). Washington, DC: Center for Global Development.

Finnemore, M., & Sikkink, K. (1998). International norm dynamics and political change. *International Organization, 52*(4), 887–917.

Freire, P. (1970). *Pedagogy of the oppressed* (M. B. Ramos, trans.). New York, NY: Seabury.

Fullan, M. (1989). *Implementing education change: What do we know?* Washington, DC: World Bank.

Gajanayake, S. (1992). *Non-formal primary education program: Mid-term evaluation*. Dhaka, Bangladesh: BRAC Donor Liaison Office.

Georgiou, G., Das, J. P., & Hayward, D. (2008). Comparing the contribution of two tasks of working memory to reading in relation to phonological awareness and rapid naming speed. *Journal of Research in Reading, 31*, 302–318.

Gish, O. (1982). Selective primary health care: Old wine in new bottles. *Social Science and Medicine, 16*(6), 1049–1055.

Glewwe, P., & Zhao, M. (2006). Attaining universal primary education by 2015: An evaluation of cost-estimates. In J. E. Cohen, D. E. Bloom, & M. B. Malin (Eds.), *Educating all children: A global agenda* (pp. 415–454). Cambridge, MA: American Association of Arts and Sciences & Massachusetts Institute of Technology.

Gove, A. (2009). *Early Grade Reading Assessment toolkit.* Research Triangle Park, NC: Research Triangle Institute, and Washington, DC: World Bank.

Gove, A., & Cvelich, P. (2010). *Early reading: Igniting Education for All. A report by the early grade learning community of practice.* Research Triangle Park, NC: Research Triangle Institute.

Gove, A., & Wetterberg, A. (Eds.). (2011). *Early grade reading assessment: Applications and interventions to improve basic literacy.* Research Triangle Park, NC: Research Triangle Institute.

Government of Bangladesh, Directorate of Primary Education, Primary and Mass Education Division. (1999). *Primary education in Bangladesh* (2nd ed.). Dhaka, Bangladesh: Government of Bangladesh.

Government of Bangladesh, Directorate of Primary Education, Primary and Mass Education Division. (2001). *Primary education in Bangladesh: Findings of PSPMP 2000* (occasional). Dhaka, Bangladesh: Data International Ltd with Academy for Educational Development.

Grant, J. P. (1987). Overview. In R. Cash, G. Keusch, & J. Lamstain (Eds.), *Child health and survival: The UNICEF GOBI-FFF program* (pp. 1–5). Beckenham, England: Croom Helm Ltd.

Greaney, V., Khandker, S. R., & Alam, M. (1999). *Bangladesh: Assessing basic learning skills* (Bangladesh Development Series). Dhaka, Bangladesh: University Press Limited for the World Bank.

Greenough III, W. (1985, October). *Specific public health measures. Good health at low cost* (S. B. Halstead, J. A. Walsh, & K. S. Warren, Eds.). (pp. 215–232). Bellagio, Italy: Rockefeller Foundation.

Greenough III, W. (2003). First experiences in Dacca: 1962–1965. In J. Sack & M. Karim (Eds.), *Smriti: ICDDR,B in memory* (pp. 54–55). Dhaka, Bangladesh: ICDDR,B.

Greenough III, W. (2004). The human, societal, and scientific legacy of cholera. *The Journal of Clinical Investigation, 113*(3), 334–339.

Haas, P. M. (1992, Winter). Knowledge, power, and international policy coordination. *International Organization, 46*(1), 1–35.

Hanushek, E. A., & Woessmann, L. (2007). *Education quality and economic growth.* Washington, DC: World Bank.

Hanushek, E. A., & Woessmann, L. (2009). *Do better schools lead to more growth? Cognitive skills, economic outcomes, and causation.* Washington, DC: National Bureau of Economic Research.

Hartmann, B., & Boyce, J. K. (1985). *A quiet violence: View from a Bangladesh village.* San Francisco, CA: Food First Books.

Havelock, R. G., & Huberman, A. M. (1978). *Solving educational problems: The theory and reality of innovation in developing countries.* New York, NY: Praeger.

Hirschhorn, N. (1987). Oral rehydration therapy: The program and the promise. In R. Cash, G. Keusch, & J. Lamstain (Eds.), *Child health and survival: The UNICEF GOBI-FFF program* (pp. 21–46). Beckenham, England: Croom Helm Ltd.

Hirschhorn, N. (1990, November). From bedside to worldwide: The progress of Oral Rehydration Therapy. Paper presented at the fifth annual Charles A. Dana Award for Pioneering Achievement in Health and Education, New York, NY.

Hirschman, A. O. (1968). Underdevelopment, obstacles to the perception of change, and leadership. *Daedalus, 3*, 925–937.

Hirschman, A. O. (1975). Policymaking and policy analysis in Latin America—A return journey. *Policy Sciences, 6*(4), 385–403.

Hirschman, A. O. (1984). *Getting ahead collectively: Grassroots experiences in Latin America*. New York, NY: Pergamon.

Hirschmann, D. (1999). Development management versus Third World bureaucracies: A brief history of conflicting interests. *Development and Change, 30*, 287–305.

Hoffman, J. (2012). Why EGRA—a clone of DIBELS—will fail to improve literacy in Africa. *Research in the Teaching of English, 46*(4), 340–357.

Hollingsworth, S., & Gains, P. (2009). *The systematic method for reading success (SMRS) in South Africa: A literacy intervention between EGRA pre- and post-assessments. Lessons learned from SMRS mastery tests and teacher performance checklists*. Research Triangle Park, NC: RTI International.

Hossain, M. H. (1994). *Traditional culture and modern systems: Administering primary education in Bangladesh*. Lanham, MD: University Press of America.

Illich, I. (1970). *Deschooling society*. New York, NY: Harper & Row.

Illich, I. (1976). *Medical nemesis*. London, England: Calder & Boyars.

Jain, P. S. (1997). Program success and management of integrated primary education in developing countries. *World Development, 25*(3), 349–352.

Jalaluddin, A. K., & Chowdhury, A. M. R. (Eds.). (1997). *Getting started: Universalizing quality primary education in Bangladesh* (vol. 1). Dhaka, Bangladesh: The University Press Limited.

Jang, Y. S. (2000). The worldwide founding of ministries of science and technology, 1950–1990. *Sociological Perspectives, 43*, 247–270.

Jepperson, R. L. (1991). Institutions, institutional effects, and institutionalism. In W. W. Powell & P. J. DiMaggio (Eds.), *The new institutionalism in organizational analysis* (pp. 143–163). Chicago, IL: University of Chicago Press.

Jessee, C., Mchazime, H., Dowd, A. J., Winicki, F., Harris, A., & Schubert, J. (2003). *Exploring factors that influence teaching and learning: Summary findings from the IEQ/Malawi longitudinal study 1999–2002*. Available at www.ieq.org/pdf/Exploration_into_Findings.pdf

Johnson, D., Hayter, J., & Broadfoot, P. (2000). *The quality of learning and teaching in developing countries: Assessing literacy and numeracy in Malawi and Sri Lanka*. London, England: U.K. Department for International Development.

Jones, P. (2005). *The United Nations and education: Multilateralism, development and globalisation*. New York, NY: RoutledgeFalmer.

Jones, P. W. (1990). UNESCO and the politics of global literacy. *Comparative Education Review, 34*(1), 41–60.

Khan, K., & Chowdhury, A. (1991). *Performance of former NFPE students in formal schools*. Dhaka, Bangladesh: BRAC Research and Evaluation Division.

Khan, K., & Chowdhury, A. M. R. (1993). *Identifying the reasons for dropout of former NFPE students in formal schools and Manikganj and Narshingdi.* Dhaka, Bangladesh: BRAC Research and Evaluation Division.

Khan, N., & Khan, K. (1993). *Education for freedom: The children of BRAC's urban schools.* Dhaka, Bangladesh: BRAC Research and Evaluation Division.

Khan, Z. R., & Arefeen, H. (1992). *Primary education in Bangladesh: A study of eight villages.* Dhaka, Bangladesh: Dhaka University; Washington, DC: Academy for Educational Development.

King, K. (1991). The golden fleece: The search for low-cost quality in primary education for all. In K. King, *Aid and education in the developing world: The role of the donor agencies in educational analysis* (pp. 195–238). London, England: Longman.

Klees, S. J. (2012). Reading mania. Education in crisis: Monitoring, analyses and resources for education activities. Available at www.educationincrisis.net/blog/item/552-reading-mania

Klouda, A. (1983). "Prevention" is more costly than "cure": Health problems for Tanzania, 1971–81. In D. Morley, J. Rohde, & G. Williams (Eds.), *Practicing health for all* (pp. 49–63). New York, NY: Oxford University Press.

Klouda, A. (1993). Prevention is *still* more costly than cure. In J. Rohde, M. Chatterjee, & D. Morley (Eds.), *Reaching Health for All* (pp. 10–27). New York, NY: Oxford University Press.

Korten, D. C. (1980, September/October). Community organization and rural development: A learning process approach. *Public Administration Review, 32,* 480–512.

Korten, D. C. (1984). Rural development programming: The learning-process approach. In D. C. Korten & R. Klaus (Eds.), *People-centered development.* West Hartford, CT: Kumarian.

Korten, D. C. (1989). *Transforming a bureaucracy: The experience of the Philippine national irrigation administration.* West Hartford, CT: Kumarian.

Krucken, G., & Drori, G. (Eds.). (2009). *World society: The writings of John W. Meyer.* Oxford, England: Oxford University Press.

Kuhn, T. S. (1996). *The structure of scientific revolutions* (3rd ed.). Chicago: University of Chicago Press. (Original work published 1962)

Laugharn, P. A. (2001). Negotiating "education for many": Enrollment, dropout, and persistence in the community schools of Kolondièba, Mali. Unpublished doctoral dissertation, University of London.

Le Boterf, G. (1984). The challenge of mass education in Nicaragua. *Assignment Children: Going to Scale for Child Survival and Development, 65/68,* 247–266.

Letshabo, K. (2002). *Technical evaluation of breakthrough to literacy in Uganda.* Kampala, Uganda: UNICEF.

Lewin, K. (1958). *Group decision and social change.* New York, NY: Holt, Rinehart, and Winston.

Lewin, K. M., & Stuart, J. (Eds.). (1991). *Educational innovation in developing countries: Case studies of changemakers.* London, England: Macmillan.

Lewis, D. (2007). *The management of non-governmental organizations* (2nd ed.). London, England: Routledge.

Lipkin, M. (1982). Selective primary health care: Commentary on critiques. *Social Science and Medicine, 16*, 1062–1064.

Lipson, M., & Wixson, K. K. (2004). *Evaluation of BTL and ASTEP programmes in the Northern, Eastern, and Volta regions.* Accra, Ghana: USAID.

Litsios, S. (2002). The politics of the World Health Organization. The long and difficult road to Alma-Ata: A personal reflection. *International Journal of Health Services, 32*(4), 709–732.

Litsios, S. (2004). The Christian Medical Commission and the development of the World Health Organization's primary health care approach. *American Journal of Public Health, 94*(11), 1884–1893.

Little, A., Hoppers, W., & Gardner, R. (Eds.). (1994). *Beyond Jomtien: Implementing primary education for all.* London, England: Macmillan.

Lockheed, M., & Verspoor, A. (1991). *Improving primary education in developing countries.* Oxford, England: Oxford University Press.

Loomis, S. A. (1976). *Bangladesh.* Washington, DC: U.S. Department of Public Health.

Lovell, C. (1992). *Breaking the cycle of poverty: The BRAC strategy.* Hartford, CT: Kumarian.

Lovell, C., & Abed, F. H. (1993). Scaling up in health: Two decades of learning in Bangladesh. In J. Rohde, M. Chatterjee, & D. Morley (Eds.), *Reaching Health for All* (pp. 212–238). New York, NY: Oxford University Press.

Lovell, C. H., & Fatema, K. (1989). *The BRAC Non-Formal Primary Education Programme in Bangladesh* (Assignment Children). New York, NY: UNICEF.

Lynch, J., Modgil, C., & Modgil, S. (Eds.). (1997). *Innovations in delivering primary education* (vol. 3). Herndon, VA: Cassell.

Madon, T., Hofman, K. J., Kupfer, L., & Glass, R. I. (2007, December 14). Implementation science. *Science, 318,* 1728–1729.

Mahalanabis, D. (2009). Miracle cure for an old scourge. *Bulletin of the World Health Organization, 87*(2), 92.

Mahalanabis, D., Choudhury, A. B., Bagchi, N. G., Bhattacharya, A. K., & Simpson, T. W. (1973). Oral fluid therapy of cholera among Bangladeshi refugees. *Johns Hopkins Medical Journal, 132,* 197–205.

Mannan, M., Chowdhury, A., & Karim, F. (1994). *Fatwabaz against BRAC: Are they alone?* Dhaka, Bangladesh: BRAC Research and Evaluation Division.

Marshall, G. (Ed.). (1994). *The concise dictionary of sociology.* New York, NY: Oxford University.

McEwan, P. J. (2013). Improving learning in primary schools of developing countries: A meta-analysis of randomized experiments. Unpublished manuscript, Wellesley, MA.

McGrane, S. (2003). A simple solution: How a healthy dose of scientific competition led to oral rehydration therapy, which saves millions of children's lives every year [Electronic Version]. Johns Hopkins Public Health. Available at magazine. jhsph.edu/2003/spring/prologue/

Meyer, J. W. (1977). The effects of education as an institution. *American Journal of Sociology, 63*, 55–77.

Meyer, J. W., Boli, J., Thomas, G. M., & Ramirez, F. O. (1997). World society and the nation state. *American Journal of Sociology, 103*(1), 144–181.

Miske, S. (2003). *Proud pioneers: Malawian teachers implement continuous assessment in primary school classrooms.* Washington, DC: American Institutes of Research.

Moats, L. C. (1999). *Teaching reading is rocket science: What expert teachers of reading should know and be able to do.* Washington, DC: American Federation of Teachers.

Mohsin, M. (1992). *Literacy in rural Bangladesh: Enrollment and dropout in selected NFPE villages.* Dhaka, Bangladesh: BRAC Research and Evaluation Division.

Mohsin, M., Nath, S. R., & Chowdhury, A. M. R. (1994). Basic competencies of children in Bangladesh: An analysis of rural/urban differential. *Pakistan Economic and Social Review, 32*(i), 61–77.

Molla, M. S. R. (2005). *Corruption in primary education in Bangladesh: TIB analysis and initiatives* (PowerPoint presentation). Dhaka, Bangladesh: Transparency International Bangladesh.

Morley, D., Rohde, J., & Williams, G. (Eds.). (1983). *Practicing Health for All.* New York, NY: Oxford University Press.

Mosley, W. (2003). The Pak-SEATO Cholera Research Laboratory. In J. Sack & M. Rahim (Eds.), *Smriti: ICDDR,B in memory* (pp. 58–60). Dhaka, Bangladesh: ICDDR,B.

Mosteller, F., & Boruch, R. (Eds.). (2002). *Evidence matters: Randomized trials in education research.* Washington, DC: Brookings Institution.

Moulton, J., Rawley, C., & Sedere, U. (2002). *NGOs as deliverers of basic education* (Bangladesh Education Sector Review Report No. 3). Washington, DC: USAID and GroundWork, Inc.

Munari, A. (1994). Jean Piaget (1896-1980). *Prospects, the quarterly review of comparative education, XXIV*(1/2), 311–327.

Naik, C. (1980). An action-research project on universal primary education: Maharashtra state, India. *Assignment Children, 51/52*, 93–113.

Nalin, D. R. (2003). Reminiscence on the development of ORS. In J. Sack & M. Karim (Eds.), *Smriti: ICDDR,B in memory* (pp. 87–89). Dhaka, Bangladesh: ICDDR,B.

Nath, S. (2000). *Basic competencies of the graduates of BRAC's non-formal schools: Levels and trends from 1995 to 1999.* Dhaka, Bangladesh: BRAC Research and Evaluation Division.

Nath, S. (2006). *Achievement of primary competencies: A comparison between government and BRAC schools.* Dhaka, Bangladesh: BRAC Research and Evaluation Division.

Nath, S., & Chowdhury, A. M. R. (1996). *Assessment of basic competencies of the graduates of BRAC's education program.* Dhaka, Bangladesh: BRAC Research and Evaluation Division.

Nath, S., Khan, K. A., & Chowdhury, A. M. R. (1994). *Progress in basic competencies of NFPE and PEOC graduates over time*. Dhaka, Bangladesh: BRAC Research and Evaluation Division. National Center for Education Statistics. (2013). California grade 4 reading: 2013 state snapshot report. *The nation's report card*. Washington, DC: U.S. Department of Education. Available at nces.ed.gov/nationsreportcard/subject/publications/stt2013/pdf/2014464CA4.pdf

Nath, S., Mohsin, M., & Chowdhury, A. (1992). *Assessment of basic education of NFPE and PEOC graduates*. Dhaka: BRAC Research and Evaluation Division.

National Research Council. (2002). *Scientific research in education* (Committee on Scientific Principles for Education Research). Washington, DC: National Academy Press.

National Research Council. (2004). *Implementing randomized field trials in education: Report of a workshop* (Committee on Research in Education). Washington, DC: National Academies Press.

Nelson, C. (1985, revised). Collaborative research on tropical diseases. In Steering Committee for the Study of U.S. Capacity to Address Tropical Infectious Disease Problem, Board on Science and Technology for International Development, National Research Council (Ed.), *The U.S. capacity to address tropical infectious disease problems*. Washington, DC: National Academy Press.

Newell, K. (1975). *Health by the people*. Geneva, Switzerland: World Health Organization.

Nielsen, H. D., & Cummings, W. K. (1999). The impact of IMPACT: A study of the dissemination of an educational innovation in six countries. In N. P. Stromquist & M. L. Basile (Eds.), *Politics of educational innovations in developing countries: An analysis of knowledge and power* (pp. 111–140). New York, NY: Falmer.

Northrup, R. (1993). Oral Rehydration Therapy: From principle to practice. In J. Rohde, M. Chatterjee, & D. Morley, (Eds.), *Reaching Health for All* (pp. 423–456). New York, NY: Oxford University Press.

Nyi Nyi. (1983). Planning, implementation and monitoring of literacy programmes: The Burmese experience. *Assignment Children, 63/64*, 87–99.

Nyi Nyi. (2001). Building foundations for the castles in the air. In R. Jolly (Ed.), *Jim Grant: UNICEF visionary* (pp. 67–86). Florence, Italy: UNICEF Innocenti Research Centre.

Organisation for Economic Co-operation and Development, Centre for Educational Research and Innovation. (1973). *Strategies for innovation in education*. Washington, DC: OECD Publication Center.

Pritchett, L. (2001). Where has all the education gone? *World Bank Economic Review, 15*(3), 367–392.

Psacharopoulos, G., & Woodhall, M. (1985). *Education for development: An analysis of investment choices*. New York, NY: Oxford University Press.

Quotah, E. (1999). Cholera: A not so simple solution. *Harvard School of Public Health Review*. Available at www.hsph.harvard.edu/review/summer_solution.shtml

Racelis, M. (2001). Controversy and continuity: Programming for women in Jim

Grant's UNICEF. In R. Jolly (Ed.), *Jim Grant: UNICEF visionary* (pp. 111–135). Florence, Italy: UNICEF Innocenti Research Center.

Rahman, M. (1994, February). *ORS in Matlab.* Paper presented at the Conference Celebrating 25 Years of ORS, Dhaka, Bangladesh. Reproduced in J. Sack & M. Rahim (Eds.), *Smriti: ICDDR,B in memory* (p. 92). Dhaka, Bangladesh: ICDDR,B.

Rahman Rahman Huq. (1992). *Cost comparison of BRAC NFP and government primary schools* (Final No. 1). Dhaka, Bangladesh: Academy for Educational Development.

Ramirez, F. O. (2012). The world society perspective: Concepts, assumptions, and strategies. *Comparative Education, 48*(4), 423–439.

Ramirez, F. O., & Boli, J. (1987). Global patterns of educational institutionalization. In G. Thomas, J. W. Meyer, F. O. Ramirez, & J. Boli (Eds.), *Institutional structure: Constituting state, society, and the individual* (pp. 150–172). Newbury Park, CA: Sage.

Rashid, S., & Chowdhury, A. (1994). *An inside look at two BRAC schools in Matlab thana.* Dhaka, Bangladesh: BRAC.

Research Triangle Institute International & International Rescue Committee. (2012). *Guidance notes for planning and implementing EGRA.* Washington, DC: Authors.

Riddell, A. (2011). Bangladesh. In A. Riddell (Ed.), *Donors and capacity development in Guyana and Bangladesh* (pp. 41–58). Paris, France: UNESCO and the International Institute for Educational Planning.

Rockefeller Foundation. (1985, October). *Good health at low cost* (S. B. Halstead, J. A. Walsh and K. S. Warren, Eds.). Bellagio, Italy: Author.

Rogers, E. M. (2003). *Diffusion of innovations* (5th ed.). New York, NY: Free Press.

Rogers, E. M., & Shoemaker, F. F. (1971). *Communication of innovations: A cross-cultural approach* (2nd ed.). New York, NY: Free Press.

Rohde, C. (2014). Catalyst: In the wake of the great Bhola cyclone. Available at CreateSpace Independent Publishing Platform.

Rohde, J. E. (1982, March 15). *Why the other half dies: The science and politics of child mortality in the Third World* (The Leonard Parsons Memorial Lecture, University of Birmingham, U.K.). Paris, France: UNESCO Unit for Co-operation with UNICEF and World Food Programme.

Rohde, J. E. (2005a). How and what BRAC learns in health: An overview. In J. E. Rohde (Ed.), *Learning to reach Health for All: Thirty years of instructive experience at BRAC* (pp. 1–32). Dhaka, Bangladesh: University Press Limited.

Rohde, J. E. (2005b). Timeline of BRAC health programmes: Major innovations and activities. In J. E. Rohde (Ed.), *Learning to reach Health for All: Thirty years of instructive experience at BRAC* (pp. xvii–xx). Dhaka, Bangladesh: University Press Limited.

Rohde, J. E. (Ed.). (2005c). *Learning to reach Health for All: Thirty years of instructive experience at BRAC.* Dhaka, Bangladesh: University Press Limited.

Rohde, J. E., & Northrup, R. S. (1976). *Taking science where the diarrhea is.* Paper presented at the Conference on Acute Diarrhea in Childhood, Amsterdam, CIBA Foundation Symposium No. 46 (CIBA Foundation, Ed.; pp. 336–339). Available at www.popline.org/node/450357

Rondinelli, D. (1976). International requirements for project preparation: Aids or obstacles to development planning? *Journal of the American Institute of Planners, 42*(3), 343.

Roskos, K., Strickland, D., Haase, J., & Malik, S. (2009). *First principles for early grades reading programs in developing countries.* Washington, DC: American Institutes for Research and U.S. Agency for International Development.

Royer, J. M., Abadzi, H., & Kinda, J. (2004). The impact of phonological awareness and rapid-reading training on the reading skills of adolescent and adult neo-literates. *International Review of Education, 50*(1), 53–72.

Rugh, A., & Bossert, H. (1998). *Involving communities: Participation in the delivery of education programs.* Washington, DC: Creative Associates International (with funds from ABEL2).

Russell, J. M., & Hirschhorn, N. (1987). For want of a nail: The problems of implementation: A national oral rehydration program. In R. Cash, G. Keusch, & J. Lamstain (Eds.), *Child health and survival: The UNICEF GOBI-FFF program* (pp. 233–239). Beckenham, England: Croom Helm Ltd.

Ruxin, J. (1994). Magic bullet: The history of Oral Rehydration Therapy. *Medical History, 38,* 363–397.

Sack, R. B. (2003). History of the development of oral rehydration fluids. *Journal of Indian Medical Association, 101*(6), 360–364.

Sack, J., & Karim, M. (Eds.). (2003). *Smriti: ICDDR,B in memory.* Dhaka, Bangladesh: ICDDR,B.

Samoff, J., Sebatane, E. M., & Dembele, M. (2005, September). "Going to scale": Nurturing the local roots of education innovation in Africa. Paper presented at the Oxford International Conference on Education and Development, Oxford, England.

Santosham, M., Keenan, E. M., Jim, T., Broun, D., & Glass, R. (1997). Oral rehydration therapy for diarrhea: An example of reverse transfer of technology. *Pediatrics, 100*(5), 10–12.

Schultz, T. W. (1961). Investment in human capital. *American Economic Review, 51,* 1–16.

Schultz, T. W. (1993). The economic importance of human capital in modernization. *Education Economics, 1*(1), 13.

Schwartz, A. (2011). *Remedial education programs to accelerate learning for all* (third draft manuscript). Washington, DC: EFA Fast Track Initiative.

Scrimshaw, N. S. (1987). Summarising the UNICEF conference on child health and survival: A personal opinion. In R. Cash, G. Keusch, & J. Lamstain (Eds.), *Child health and survival: The UNICEF GOBI-FFF program* (pp. 244–250). Beckenham, England: Croom Helm Ltd.

Sedere, M. U. (1995). *Non-formal primary education program (NFPE): Lessons to learn* (General Education Project Working Papers). Dhaka, Bangladesh: World Bank Resident Mission.

Seidel, R. (2005). *Behavior change perspectives and communication guidelines on six Child Survival interventions.* Geneva, Switzerland and New York, NY: Family Health International.

Share, D. L. (2008). On the Anglocentricities of current reading research and practice: The perils of overreliance on an "outlier" orthography. *Psychological Bulletin, 134*(4), 584–615.

Shordt, K. (1991). *The expansion of BRAC's Non-Formal Primary Education program, 1990–1992.* Dhaka, Bangladesh: BRAC Donor Liaison Office.

Siddique, A. (2003). Innovations saved lives: The untold story of Goma. In J. Sack & M. Rahim (Eds.), *Smriti: ICDDR,B in memory* (pp. 124–126). Dhaka, Bangladesh: ICDDR,B

Siddique, A., Salam, A., Islam, M., Akram, K., Majumdar, R., Zaman, K., et al. (1995). Why treatment centres failed to prevent cholera deaths among Rwandan refugees in Goma, Zaire. *Lancet, 345*(8946), 124–126.

Smillie, I. (2009). *Freedom from want: The remarkable success story of BRAC, the global grassroots organization that's winning the fight against poverty.* Sterling, VA: Kumarian.

Stein, H. D. (2007). *UNICEF in Bellagio: A memoir.* New York, NY: UNICEF.

Stigler, J. (1999). *The TIMSS videotape classroom study: Methods and findings from an exploratory research project on eighth-grade mathematics instruction in Germany, Japan, and the United States.* Washington, DC: U.S. Department of Education, Office of Educational Research and Improvement, National Center for Education Statistics.

Stokes, D. E. (1997). *Pasteur's quadrant: Basic science and technological innovation.* Washington, DC: Brookings Institution.

Stromquist, N. P., & Basile, M. L. (Eds.). (1999). *Politics of educational innovations in developing countries: An analysis of knowledge and power* (vol. 46). New York: Falmer.

Strand, D., & Meyer, J. W. (2009). Diffusion: Institutional conditions for diffusion. In G. Krucken & G. Drori (Eds.), *World society: The writing of John W. Meyer* (pp. 136–155). Oxford, England: Oxford University Press. (Original work published 1993)

Suarez, D. (2007). Education professionals and the construction of human rights education. *Comparative Education Review, 51,* 48–70.

Sunoto, S., Budiarso, A. D., & Wiharta, A. S. (1983). Sugar-salt solution using standard plastic scoops: Blue spoon in the treatment of acute diarrhea. *Paediatrica Indonesiana, 23*(11–12), 227–229.

Sweetser, A. T. (1999). *Lessons from the BRAC Non-Formal Primary Education program.* Washington, DC: Academy for Education Development and USAID.

Taylor, C., & Bryant, J. (2008, May 24). The Christian community's contribution to the evolution of community-based primary health care. Paper presented at the annual conference of Christian Connections for International Health (CCIH).

Thomas, G. M., Meyer, J. W., Ramirez, F. O., & Boli, J. (1987). *Institutional structure: Constituting state, society, and the individual.* Newbury Park, CA: Sage.

Tietjen, K., Rahman, A., & Spaulding, S. (2004). *Time to learn: Teachers' and students' use of time in government primary schools in Bangladesh* (Bangladesh Educational Assessment for USAID/Dhaka). Washington, DC: Creative Associates Inc.

Torgerson, C. J., & Torgerson, D. J. (2003). The design and conduct of randomised controlled trials in education: Lessons from health care. *Oxford Review of Education, 29*(1), 67–80.

Tudor, A. (2007). Induction and observation in science. Available at www.sociology-encyclopedia.com

UNESCO. (2000a, April). Assessing learning achievement. Paper presented at the World Education Forum, Dakar, Senegal.

UNESCO. (2000b, April). Final report. Paper presented at the World Education Forum, Dakar, Senegal.

UNESCO-UNICEF Cooperative Programme. (1978). *Basic services for children: A continuing search for learning priorities. A dossier for initiating a dialogue: Part I* (No. 36 & 37). Geneva, Switzerland: International Bureau of Education.

United Nations Children's Fund. (1987). *An analysis of the situation of children in Bangladesh.* Dhaka, Bangladesh: BRAC Press.

Unterhalter, E., Ross, J., & Alam, M. (2003). A fragile dialogue: Research and primary education policy formation in Bangladesh, 1971–2001. *Compare, 33*(1), 85–99.

Uvin, P., Jain, P. S., & Brown, L. D. (2000). Think large and act small: Toward a new paradigm for NGO scaling up. *World Development, 28*(8), 1409–1430.

van Heyningen, W. E., & Seal, J. R. (1983). *Cholera: The American scientific experience, 1947–1980.* Boulder, CO: Westview.

Vandemoortele, J. (2011). If not the Millennium Development Goals, then what? *Third World Quarterly, 32*(1), 9–26.

Varma, A., & Malviya, A. (1996). *Daunting challenge: An alternative strategy for effective delivery of primary education.* New Delhi, India: Oxfam America Inc.

Venediktov, D. (1998). Alma-Ata and after. *World Health Forum, 19,* 79–87.

Verspoor, A. (1993). More than business-as-usual: Reflections on the new modalities of education aid. *International Journal of Educational Development, 13*(2), 103–112.

Wagner, D. A. (2011). *Smaller, quicker, cheaper: Better learning assessments for developing countries.* Paris, France: UNESCO; Philadelphia, PA: International Literacy Institute.

Wahed, M. (2003). After ORS success, a struggle with acceptance. In J. Sack & M. A. Rahim (Eds.), *Smriti: ICDDR,B in memory* (p. 93). Dhaka, Bangladesh: ICDDR,B.

Walsh, J. A., & Warren, K. S. (1979). Selective primary health care: An interim strategy for disease control in developing countries. *New England Journal of Medicine, 301*(18), 967–975.

Weiss, C. H. (2002). What to do until the random assigner comes. In F. Mosteller & R. Boruch (Eds.), *Evidence matters: Randomized trials in education research* (pp. 198–224). Washington, DC: Brookings Institution.

Wejnert, B. (2002). Integrating models of diffusion of innovations: A conceptual framework. *Annual Review of Sociology, 28,* 297–336.

Werner, D. (1983). Health care in Cuba: A model service or a means of social control—or both? In D. Morley, J. Rohde, & G. Williams (Eds.), *Practising Health for All* (pp. 17–37). New York, NY: Oxford University Press.

Williams, E. (1998). *Investigating bilingual literacy: Evidence from Malawi and Zambia.* London, England: UK Department for International Development.

Windham, D. M. (1988). Indicators of educational effectiveness and efficiency (occasional). Washington, DC: Improving the Efficiency of Educational Systems Project. USAID Contract No. DPE-5283-C-00-4013-00.

Windham, D. M. (1992). Education for All: The requirements (World Conference on Education for All Monograph No. III). Paris, France: UNESCO.

Wolf, J., Kane, E., & Strickland, B. (1997). Planning for community participation in education (ABEL Technical Paper No. 1). Washington, DC: USAID.

World Bank, Human Development Sector, South Asia Region. (2013). *Bangladesh education sector review: Seeding fertile ground: Education that works for Bangladesh.* Washington, DC: World Bank.

World Bank, Independent Evaluation Group. (2006). *From schooling access to learning outcomes: An unfinished agenda. An evaluation of World Bank support to primary education* (evaluation). Washington, DC: World Bank.

World Conference on Education for All. (1990, March). World Declaration on Education for All. World Conference on Education for All, Jomtien, Thailand.

World Council of Churches. (n.d.). *Christian Medical Commission Archives: Guide to the microfilm collection.* Leiden, Netherlands: Brill, Kenneth Scott Latourette Fund and Yale Divinity School Library.

World Health Organization. (1988). *From Alma-Ata to the year 2000: Reflections at the midpoint* (Archival: National Reference Center for Bioethics Literature, Kennedy Institute, Georgetown University). Geneva, Switzerland: World Health Organization.

World Health Organization. (2008a, October). Primary health care comes full circle: An interview with Halfdan Mahler. *Bulletin of the World Health Organization, 86,* 747–748.

World Health Organization. (2008b). *World Health Report 2008: Primary health care (now more than ever).* Geneva, Switzerland: Author.

Zaman, S., & Karim, R. (2005). History of BRAC health interventions: Experience and learning. In J. Rohde (Ed.), *Learning to reach Health for All: Thirty years of instructive experience at BRAC* (pp. 33–169). Dhaka, Bangladesh: University Press Limited.

Ziegler, J., & Goswami, U. (2005). Reading acquisition, developmental dyslexia, and skilled reading across languages: A psycholinguistic grain size theory. *Psychological Bulletin, 131*(1), 3–29.

Index

About the Authors

Dr. Colette Chabbott is adjunct faculty in the International Education Program at the Graduate School of Education and Human Development at George Washington University, Washington, DC. There she teaches and writes about the sociology of international development organizations and education in Islamic Asia.

Since 1990 she has worked with several international organizations—including the William and Flora Hewlett Foundation, the Research Triangle Institute, the American Institutes for Research, UNICEF, the Consultative Group for Early Childhood Care and Education, CARE, Save the Children, and BRAC—on improving the quality of primary education in South Asia (1989–present). She worked in Egypt (1997–1998) and Yemen (2006) on issues relating to girls' education, early grades reading, social mobilization, and community schools.

Previously she served as the staff director of the Board of International Comparative Studies in Education at the (U.S.) National Research Council (2000–2003), as director of the international comparative education master's program at Stanford University (1996–1999), and as a special projects officer with USAID (1984–1992).

She earned a B.A. in economics from the University of North Carolina at Chapel Hill, an M.P.A. in development policy from the Woodrow Wilson School at Princeton University, and an A.M. in sociology and a Ph.D. in education from Stanford University. Her previous publications include *Constructing Education for Development: International Organizations and Education for All* (2003).

Dr. Mushtaque Chowdhury is the vice chairperson and interim executive director of BRAC. He is also the advisor to BRAC's founder and chairperson, Fazle Hasan Abed. Previously he was the founding director of the BRAC Research and Evaluation Division and the founding dean of the James P. Grant School of Public Health at BRAC University.

He is also a professor of population and family health at the Mailman School of Public Health of Columbia University, New York. During 2009–2012, he worked as a senior advisor to the Rockefeller Foundation, based in Bangkok, Thailand. He also served as a MacArthur Fellow at Harvard University.

Dr. Chowdhury is a founder of the Bangladesh Education Watch and Bangladesh Health Watch, two civil society watchdogs on education and health, respectively. He was a coordinator of the U.N. Millennium Task Force on Child Health and Maternal Health, set up by the former Secretary-General Kofi Annan.

He holds a Ph.D. from the London School of Hygiene and Tropical Medicine, an M.Sc. from the London School of Economics, and a B.A. from the University of Dhaka.